COVID-19 Studies Concerning Health, Social and Economic Aspects

Mustafa Demirkıran / Burhanettin Uysal (eds.)

COVID-19 Studies Concerning Health, Social and Economic Aspects

PETER LANG

**Bibliographic Information published by the
Deutsche Nationalbibliothek**
The Deutsche Nationalbibliothek lists this publication in the Deutsche
Nationalbibliografie; detailed bibliographic data is available online at
http://dnb.d-nb.de.

Library of Congress Cataloging-in-Publication Data
A CIP catalog record for this book has been applied for at the
Library of Congress.

Cover illustration: © wildpixel/istockphoto.com

ISBN 978-3-631-84112-9 (Print)
E-ISBN 978-3-631-84265-2 (E-PDF)
E-ISBN 978-3-631-84266-9 (EPUB)
E-ISBN 978-3-631-84267-6 (MOBI)
DOI 10.3726/b17876

© Peter Lang GmbH
Internationaler Verlag der Wissenschaften
Berlin 2020
All rights reserved.

Peter Lang – Berlin · Bern · Bruxelles · New York · Oxford · Warszawa · Wien

This publication has been peer reviewed.

www.peterlang.com

Table of Contents

List of Contributors

Alptuğ Aksoy
Res. Asst.; Osmaniye Korkut Ata University, Social Sciences Institute, Business Administration Program, Turkey.
alptugaksoy@osmaniye.edu.tr

Semih Baş
Lecturer; Harran University, Siverek Vocational School, Department of Medical Documentation and Secretarial, Turkey.
bas_semih@harran.edu.tr

Eylem Bayrakçı
Asst. Prof.; Isparta University of Applied Sciences, Büyükkutlu Faculty of Applied Sciences, Department of International Trade and Business, Turkey.
eylembayrakci@isparta.edu.tr

Mustafa Demirkıran
Assoc. Prof.; Isparta University of Applied Sciences, Isparta Vocational School, Department of Management and Organization, Turkey.
mustafademirkiran@isparta.edu.tr

Mehmet Dinç
Asst. Prof.; Isparta University of Applied Sciences, Büyükkutlu Faculty of Applied Sciences, Department of Accounting and Financial Management, Türkiye.
mehmetdinc@isparta.edu.tr

Hüseyin Başar Önem
Asst. Prof.; Isparta University of Applied Sciences, Isparta Vocational School, Finance Banking and Insurance Department, Turkey.
basaronem@isparta.edu.tr

Umut Can Öztürk
Asst. Prof.; Isparta University of Applied Sciences, Isparta Vocational School, Department of Management and Organization, Turkey.
umutcn.ozturk@gmail.com

Elvan Öztürk
PhD.; Turkey.
elvannozturk@gmail.com

Serap Taşkaya
Asst. Prof.; Osmaniye Korkut Ata University, Faculty of Health Science, Department of Health Care Management, Turkey.
seraptaskaya@yahoo.com

Ebrar Ulusinan
Res. Asst.; Bilecik Şeyh Edebali University, Faculty of Health Sciences, Healthcare Management Department, Turkey.
ebrar.ulusinan@bilecik.edu.tr

Burhanettin Uysal
Asst. Prof.; Bilecik Şeyh Edebali University, Faculty of Health Sciences, Healthcare Management Department, Turkey.
burhanettin.uysal@bilecik.edu.tr

Lecturer Semih Baş and Assoc. Prof. Mustafa Demirkıran

Examination of the Healthcare Institution Preferences of Individuals during COVID-19 Pandemic

1. Introduction

Coronaviruses (CoV) are one of the two members of the Coronaviridae group (Siddell, 1995) with enveloped, positive single-stranded viruses and the largest known Ribonucleic Acid (RNA) genomes (Lai & Cavanagh, 1997; Weiss & Leibowitz, 2011). Of the coronaviruses that are divided into four groups, Alpha and Beta coronaviruses are known to infect humans. The coronavirus strains that infect humans were thought not to pose a serious threat to human health (Weiss & Navas-Martin, 2005) and were generally known as coronaviruses that caused common cold (Myint, 1995). However, with the emergence of Severe acute respiratory syndrome (SARS-CoV) in 2002 and Middle East respiratory syndrome (MERS-CoV) in 2012, these two zoonotic viruses were observed to cause serious diseases and deaths (Yang & Leibowitz, 2015). According to the World Health Organization (WHO) report covering the dates of November 2002 and August 2003, 8,422 cases and 916 deaths were reported in the SARS-CoV outbreak (WHO, 2003). Regarding the MERS-CoV epidemic, the number of cases and deaths are still updated and shared by the WHO. In its 2019 status update report, the WHO reported 2,468 cases and 851 deaths from MERS between April 2012 and September 2019 (WHO, 2019).

In December 2019, new cases of pneumonia of unknown etiology appeared in the city of Wuhan in Hubei Province, China. It was determined that these cases, which were reported to be clustered in seafood market employees in Wuhan City, were caused by a new coronavirus that has not been seen in humans before (Ministry of Health of Turkey, 2020a; WHO, 2020a). Following this finding, despite the strict measures and large-scale restrictions imposed by the Chinese government, the new coronavirus reached many other countries of the world in a very short time (Fanelli & Piazza, 2020). On January 30, 2020, WHO declared the new coronavirus outbreak as a Public Health Emergency of International Concern due to 82 cases confirmed in 18 countries outside China and a total of 7,818 confirmed cases including China. According to the WHO report published on the same date, the temporary name of the disease that caused the current outbreak was proposed to be 2019-nCoV acute respiratory disease, but it was reported that the International Virus Classification Committee (ICTV) was to decide on the official name of the virus (WHO, 2020b). ICTV announced that the virus that caused the outbreak was named Severe Acute Respiratory Syndrome Coronavirus-2 (SARS-CoV-2), due to the high genetic similarity between it and the SARS virus of 2002 (Gorbalenya et al., 2020). Thereupon, WHO announced that the SARS-CoV-2 virus caused Coronavirus Disease 2019 (COVID-19) disease (WHO, 2020d).

The first COVID-19 case in Turkey was detected on March 10, 2020, and announced by the Health Minister Dr. Fahrettin Koca on March 11, 2020 (Ministry of Health of Turkey, 2020b). On the same date, WHO declared the COVID-19 disease as a Pandemic affecting the world, after more than 118,000 cases were found in 114 different countries and 4,291 people died (WHO, 2020c). As a result of the increasing cases and related deaths, the Turkish government implemented strict and comprehensive measures against the COVID-19 outbreak. With the control of the disease over time and the decrease in the number of cases and deaths, the measures have been gradually relaxed as of June 1, 2020. With the relaxation of the measures and the prohibitions' gradual lifting, the "controlled social life" style was adopted and the authorities frequently emphasized the importance of wearing a mask, social distancing, and personal hygiene during this period.

COVID-19 is a type of disease that is transmitted between humans by contact and droplet (Sabino-Silva et al., 2020) and has no specific treatment with proven efficacy and validity (Chen et al., 2020; Lai et al., 2020; Murthy et al., 2020). There is no approved drug/s used to cure the COVID-19, and no results have been gotten regarding vaccination studies yet (Shaw et al., 2020). In the literature, studies and scientific publications related to the status of alternative treatments are ongoing (Tillu et al., 2020; Uysal & Ulusinan, 2020). The Center for Disease Control and Prevention described the symptoms as fever, dry cough, shortness of breath, fatigue, muscle and joint pain, loss of taste and smell, sore throat, diarrhea, nausea and vomiting, and nasal congestion or runny nose. The organization also stated that these symptoms appeared 2 to 14 days after exposure to the virus. Individuals who have no symptoms despite carrying the SARS-CoV-2 virus that causes COVID-19 and individuals with the disease in the incubation period can transmit the virus to others they come into contact with (Gu et al., 2020).

Hospitals and other healthcare institutions are cited as places where the risk of transmission of the COVID-19 pandemic is high (Kamps & Hoffmann, 2020). Intensive filling of hospitals by infected patients increases the risk of transmission of the virus to healthcare personnel and other uninfected patients (Nacoti et al., 2020). This situation may cause the individuals to either postpone their right to use healthcare services, which is defined as the most fundamental right (Kılıç & Çalışkan, 2013), or to turn to healthcare institutions where they think the risk of virus transmission is lower.

Examination of the demand for healthcare services contributes to the efficient administration of the healthcare sector (Saraçoğlu & Öztürk, 2016; Naldöken et al., 2018). Especially during the COVID-19 Pandemic, we are experiencing, examining the demand for healthcare services is of great importance for planning healthcare services and the health sector to effectively fight the pandemic.

Demands for healthcare services also make up the supply of healthcare services (Aydın, 2008). The supply of curative health services is provided by primary, secondary, and tertiary therapeutic health services (Olesen & Fleming, 1998; Ministry of Health of Turkey, 2019).

The family physician, who is responsible for the supply of primary health care services, is defined as a family medicine specialist who is responsible for providing personalized preventive health services as well as primary care diagnosis, treatment, and rehabilitative health services, or a specialist physician or general practitioner who has received the training prescribed by the Ministry of Health of Turkey (Family Medicine Law, 2004: Article 2). The place where one or more family physicians come together to provide healthcare services accompanied by other health personnel is called a family health center (Kavuncubaşı & Yıldırım, 2015).

Secondary healthcare services are provided by public and private hospitals known as inpatient treatment institutions. Hospitals are defined as institutions where the sick and injured, those who suspect of illnesses and those who want to have their health status checked, are observed, examined, diagnosed, treated, and rehabilitated on an outpatient or inpatient basis, and also give birth (Inpatient Treatment Institutions Management Regulation, 1983: Article 4).

The supply of tertiary healthcare services is provided by university hospitals and training and research hospitals. The main purpose of such healthcare institutions is to train health professionals and to carry out fully equipped and comprehensive treatment services (Ateş, 2011; Tengilimoğlu et al., 2017).

There are 7,979 Family Health Centers and 26,252 Family Medicine Units in Turkey. A total of 1,534 hospitals, consisting of 889 hospitals affiliated with the Ministry of Health, 577 hospitals affiliated with private enterprises, 68 hospitals affiliated with universities, provide secondary and tertiary health services. According to 2018 data, 782.515.204 healthcare requests were made. 33.03 %

of these requests were directed to family medicine units, 48.64 % to general hospitals affiliated with the Ministry of Health of Turkey, 5.45 % to university hospitals, 11.98 % to private medical centers and private hospitals (Ministry of Health of Turkey, 2018).

The demand for healthcare services can be defined as the state of being able to benefit from healthcare institutions and organizations in order to get information and support without any health problems (Mills & Gilson, 1998) or in case of a health problem (Yaylalı et al., 2012). The healthcare service demand of the individual arises from the desire to fill the gap between the current health status and the ideal health status (Mooney, 2003; Kavuncubaşı & Yıldırım, 2015). Factors affecting the choice of health services in the literature are examined under many different headings such as price, income level, education, transportation, time spent in the healthcare institution, health level and disease severity, availability of health insurance, quality of health services, and the role of the physician (Yaylalı et al., 2012; Saraçoğlu & Öztürk, 2016; Çelik, 2019).

This study was carried out to examine the changes in individuals' healthcare institution preferences during the COVID-19 pandemic process and determine the factors affecting these preferences. Especially during the pandemic period, considering that healthcare institutions are intensive and often crowded and confined spaces, individuals are expected to change their healthcare institution preferences.

2. Methods

The population of this study, which was carried out to examine the changes in individuals' healthcare institution preferences during the COVID-19 pandemic, and to determine the factors affecting these preferences, consists of people aged 18 and over living within the borders of Turkey. The number of people aged 18 and over in Turkey could not be determined, but according to the Turkish Statistical Institute (2019) data, the number of people aged 15 and over is 63,94 million. With a 95 % confidence interval and a 5 % margin of error, a population between 1 million and 100 million can be represented by a sample of 384 people (Yazıcıoğlu & Erdoğan, 2004).

The survey method was used to obtain the data needed for the study. There are nine (9) questions in the questionnaire created by the researchers. The first two questions are about the individuals' healthcare institution preferences before and during the pandemic period. Relevant healthcare institutions were examined under four headings: "Family Health Center," "General/ State Hospital," "Education and Research/ University Hospital" and "Private Hospital/ Private

Medical Center." The third question of the questionnaire was asked in order to measure the reasoning behind the preference of healthcare institutions of the participants during the pandemic period. Other questions of the questionnaire are questions to determine the socio-demographic characteristics of the participants.

The created questionnaire was applied between 07.09.2020–11.09.2020 by considering the pandemic and using an online survey method. The questionnaire was also shared with those who requested it, using methods such as sending it via e-mail. Between the specified dates, 536 people participated by filling out the questionnaire. Data were analyzed using appropriate statistical methods.

Approval was obtained from the Ministry of Health of Turkey in order to conduct the study. In addition, the permission of the Scientific Research and Publication Ethics Board of Isparta University of Applied Sciences, dated 07.09.2020 and numbered 2 was obtained.

3. Results

In this part of the study, findings regarding the changes in individuals' healthcare institution preferences during the COVID-19 pandemic and the factors affecting these preferences are presented. The participants' socio-demographic characteristics, the healthcare institution preferences before and during the pandemic period, the factors affecting the healthcare institution preferences during the pandemic period were compared and evaluated.

As presented in Tab. 1, most of the participants are in the 18–24 age group (40.7 %). The proportion of female participants (57.6 %) is higher than that of male participants (42.4 %). Although the marital status of the individuals participating in the study shows a balanced distribution, unmarried (53.0 %) rate is higher than the rate of married (47.0 %). While most of the participants are university graduates (68.1 %), the average monthly income of the individuals shows a balanced distribution. When the place of residence information is examined, it can be seen that the participants are concentrated in the city center (45.0 %) and the district center (%38.8).

Tab. 2 contains information about the participants' healthcare institution preferences in the pre-pandemic period and during the pandemic. According to this information, there are important differences between the healthcare institution preferences of the participants. During the pandemic period, the preference for "Private hospital/ private medical center" increased by 81 %, and the preference for "Family health center" increased by 24 %. On the other hand,

Tab. 1. Socio-demographic characteristics of the participants

Age	n	%	Place of residence	n	%
18–24	218	40,7	City center	241	45,0
25–34	100	18,7	District center	208	38,8
35–44	124	23,1	Village/ town	87	16,2
45 ve above	94	17,5	**Average income**	n	%
Gender	n	%	2500 ve below	145	27,1
Male	227	42,4	2501–4000	149	27,8
Female	309	57,6	4001–6000	118	22,0
Marital status	n	%	6001 ve above	117	21,8
Married	252	47,0	Total	529	98,7
Unmarried	284	53,0	Missing	7	1,3
Education status	n	%	**Total**	536	100,0
Primary school	68	12,7			
Secondary school	103	19,2			
University	365	68,1			

Tab. 2. Healthcare institution preferences of the participants

Healthcare institution	Healthcare institution preference in the pre-pandemic period		Healthcare institution preference in the pandemic period		Change	
	n	%	n	%	n	%
Family health center	139	25,9	170	31,7	+31	+24
General/ state hospital	245	45,7	163	30,4	-82	-33
Education and research/ university hospital	63	11,8	42	7,8	-21	-33
Private hospital/ private medical center	89	16,6	161	30,0	+72	+81
Total	536	%100	536	%100		

"Training and research/ university hospital" and "General/ state hospital" preferences show a decrease of 33 %. The information presented in the table also shows that the participants mostly preferred the "General/ state hospital" (45.7 %) in the pre-pandemic period, and the "Family health center" the most (31.7 %) during the pandemic.

Tab. 3. Factors affecting the healthcare institution preferences of participants in the pandemic process

No	Factors	Healthcare institution				Total
		Family health center (n)	General/ state hospital (n)	Training and research/ university hospital (n)	Private hospital/ private medical center (n)	
1	A lesser risk of virus transmission	41	7	3	61	112
2	Low patient density	60			44	104
3	Proximity to home	37	32	2	4	75
4	Faster execution of procedures	8	8	2	40	58
5	Greater scope of services offered		27	14	7	48
6	Greater attention devoted to patients	5		2	40	47
7	Satisfaction with the health services provided		23		11	34
8	To be generally reliable	2	18	3	5	28
9	Higher knowledge and experience of physicians		14	7	3	24
10	Financial difficulties	1	20	3		24
11	Modern devices and technological infrastructure		11	9	2	22
12	Not to occupy hospitals except for serious illnesses	20				20
13	History of a severe/chronic disease		4	4		8
14	Desire to be examined by the same physician		6	1		7
15	The fact that family physician know more about their patients	7				7
16	Satisfaction with the family physician's treatment practices	7				7
17	Feeling closer to the family physician	6				6
18	Having an acquaintance among personnel		4		2	6
19	Presence of a private health insurance				4	4
20	Shorter diagnosis time		3			3
21	A more detailed examination	3				3
22	Lack of a private hospital in close proximity to home		3			3

(continued on next page)

Tab. 3. Continued

No	Factors	Healthcare institution				
		Family health center (n)	General/ state hospital (n)	Training and research/ university hospital (n)	Private hospital/ private medical center (n)	Total
23	The belief that the correct medicine will be prescribed		2			2
24	Single patient rooms				2	2
25	Contacting fewer people	1				1
26	24/7 service availability		1			1
27	Feeling better psychologically		1			1
28	Having a good command of one's medical condition	1				1
29	The belief that no unnecessary action will be taken		1			1
Total		199	185	50	225	659

Tab. 3 includes the factors affecting the healthcare institution preferences of the participants in the pandemic process. According to this information, the most important factors affecting the participants' choice of family health center are listed as: "Low patient density" (n=60), "A lesser risk of virus transmission" (n=41), and "Proximity to home" (n=37). The most important factors affecting the participants' choice of general/ state hospital are: "Proximity to home" (n=32), "Greater scope of services offered" (n=27), and "Satisfaction with the health services provided" (n=23). The most important factors affecting the participants' choice of education and research/ university hospital are: "Greater scope of services offered" (n=14), "Modern devices and technological infrastructure" (n=9), and "Higher knowledge and experience of physicians" (n=7).

The most important factors affecting the preference of the private hospital/ private medical center, which increased by 81 % during the pandemic process, are listed as: "A lesser risk of virus transmission" (n=61), "Low patient density" (n=44), "Faster execution of procedures" (n=40), and "Greater attention devoted to patients" (n=40). When evaluated in terms of all healthcare institutions, the most important factors affecting the healthcare institution preferences of participants during the COVID-19 pandemic process are "A lesser risk of virus transmission" (n=112), "Low patient density" (n=104), and "Proximity to home" (n=75).

Tab. 4. Distribution of healthcare institution preferences of participants by gender

Healthcare institution preference in the pre-pandemic period				Healthcare institution preference in the pandemic period			
Healthcare institution	Gender		Total	Healthcare institution	Gender		Total
	Female (n)	Male (n)			Female (n)	Male (n)	
Family health center	87	52	**139**	Family health center	99	71	**170**
General/ state hospital	131	114	**245**	General/ state hospital	84	79	**163**
Education and research/ university hospital	36	27	**63**	Education and research/ university hospital	24	18	**42**
Private hospital/ private medical center	55	34	**89**	Private hospital/ private medical center	102	59	**161**
Total	**309**	**227**	**536**	**Total**	**309**	**227**	**536**

In Tab. 4, the healthcare institution preferences of the participants are presented according to their gender. According to this information, it can be seen that the general preferences of both female participants (n=131) and male participants (n=114) in the pre-pandemic period were "General/ state hospital." During the pandemic process, it can be seen, however, that the general preferences of female participants (n=102) are "Private hospital/ Private medical center," while the general preference of male participants (n=79) is "General/ state hospital." According to the information in the table, there is a transition from "General/ state hospital" and "Education and research/ university hospital" to "Private hospital/ private medical center" and "Family health center" in the healthcare institution preferences of female and male participants during the pandemic process.

Healthcare institution preferences according to the marital status of the participants are presented in Tab. 5. According to the information in the table, while the healthcare institution preferences of both married (n=113) and unmarried (n=132) participants in the pre-pandemic period were mostly "General/ state hospital," the preferences of married participants (n=80) during the pandemic period are mostly "Private hospital/ Private medical center," and unmarried participants (n=98) mostly prefer "Family health center."

Tab. 5. Distribution of healthcare institution preferences of participants by marital status

Healthcare institution preference in the pre-pandemic period				Healthcare institution preference in the pandemic period			
Healthcare institution	Marital status		Total	Healthcare institution	Marital status		Total
	Married (n)	Unmarried (n)			Married (n)	Unmarried (n)	
Family health center	55	84	139	Family health center	72	98	170
General/ state hospital	113	132	245	General/ state hospital	74	89	163
Education and research/ university hospital	35	28	63	Education and research/ university hospital	26	16	42
Private hospital/ private medical center	49	40	89	Private hospital/ private medical center	80	81	161
Total	252	284	536	Total	252	284	536

Tab. 6. Distribution of healthcare institution preferences of participants by educational status

Healthcare institution preference in the pre-pandemic period					Healthcare institution preference in the pandemic period				
Healthcare institution	Educational status*			Total	Healthcare institution	Educational status*			Total
	A (n)	B (n)	C (n)			A (n)	B (n)	C (n)	
Family health center	15	32	92	139	Family health center	22	36	112	170
General/ state hospital	38	42	165	245	General/ state hospital	25	29	109	163
Education and research/ university hospital	9	14	40	63	Education and research/ university hospital	7	12	23	42
Private hospital/ private medical center	6	15	68	89	Private hospital/ private medical center	14	26	121	161
Total	68	103	365	536	Total	68	103	365	536

*A= Primary school, B= Secondary school, C= University

In Tab. 6, healthcare institution preferences are presented according to the education level of the participants. According to the information in the table, primary school (n=38), secondary school (n=42), and university (n=165) graduates mostly preferred the same healthcare institutions in the pre-pandemic period (General/ state hospital). Although on different levels, there is a transition to "Family health center" and "Private hospital/ private medical center" in the healthcare institution choices of the primary, secondary, and university graduates during the pandemic.

Tab. 7 shows the healthcare institution preferences of the participants according to their place of residence. The healthcare institution preference of the participants residing in the city center (n=101), district center (n=104), and village/town (n=40) in the pre-pandemic period were mostly "General/ state hospital." During the pandemic, on the other hand, the healthcare institution preference of the participants residing in the city center (n=83) is mostly "Private hospital/ private medical center" and the participants residing in the district center (n= 69) and village/town (n=40) mostly prefer "Family health center."

Tab. 7. Distribution of healthcare institution preferences of participants by place of residence

Healthcare institution preference in the pre-pandemic period					Healthcare institution preference in the pandemic period				
Healthcare institution	Place of residence*			Total	Healthcare institution	Place of residence*			Total
	A (n)	B (n)	C (n)			A (n)	B (n)	C (n)	
Family health center	55	53	31	139	Family health center	61	69	40	170
General/ state hospital	101	104	40	245	General/ state hospital	70	66	27	163
Education and research/ university hospital	42	14	7	63	Education and research/ university hospital	27	12	3	42
Private hospital/ private medical center	43	37	9	89	Private hospital/ private medical center	83	61	17	161
Total	241	208	87	536	Total	241	208	87	536

*A= City center, B= District center, C= Village/ town

Tab. 8. Distribution of healthcare institution preferences of participants by income

Healthcare institution preference in the pre-pandemic period						Healthcare institution preference in the pandemic period					
Healthcare institution	Income*				Total	Healthcare institution	Income*				Total
	A (n)	B (n)	C (n)	D (n)			A (n)	B (n)	C (n)	D (n)	
Family health center	51	37	33	18	139	Family health center	65	50	33	22	170
General/ state hospital	73	67	51	48	239	General/ state hospital	52	40	41	25	158
Education and research/ university hospital	12	16	17	17	62	Education and research/ university hospital	7	13	10	11	41
Private hospital/ private medical center	9	29	17	34	89	Private hospital/ private medical center	21	46	34	59	160
Total	145	149	118	117	529	Total	145	149	118	117	529

*A= 2500 and below, B= 2501–4000, C= 4001–6000, D= 6001 and above

Tab. 8 presents the healthcare institution preferences according to the income level of the participants. In the pre-pandemic period, participants' preferences in all income groups were mostly "General/ state hospital." During the pandemic, the healthcare institution preference of low-income participants showed a transition from "General/ state hospital" to "Family health center"; There is a transition from "General/ state hospital" to "Private Hospital/ private medical center" increasing with the income level of the participants. The participants' healthcare institution preferences with the highest income are generally "Private hospital/ private medical center."

4. Discussion

In this study, the changes in healthcare institution preferences of individuals during the COVID-19 pandemic, and the factors affecting these preferences were determined. There is no study conducted and published in the literature to determine individuals' healthcare institution preferences during pandemics or the factors affecting these preferences. However, there are many studies in Turkish and international literature regarding the demand for healthcare services. This section includes the factors affecting the changes in individuals' healthcare institution preferences during the COVID-19 pandemic and comparisons with other studies in the literature regarding the demand for health services.

The most important factor affecting the participants' healthcare institution choices of during the COVID-19 pandemic is the "A lesser risk of virus transmission" factor. In line with this information, individuals will prefer the healthcare institution that they think has a lower risk of virus transmission while choosing a healthcare institution during a pandemic. Other important factors affecting the healthcare institution choices of the participants during the COVID-19 pandemic process are listed as "Low patient density," "Proximity to home," "Faster execution of procedures." When these factors are examined, it can be seen that individuals want to minimize the risk of virus transmission while making their healthcare institution choices. The high risk of transmission of the virus in crowded environments is effective for individuals to prefer low-intensity healthcare institutions. Likewise, individuals want to minimize the risk of virus transmission by choosing a health facility close to home, avoiding public transportation, and entering crowded environments. The fact that hospitals and other healthcare institutions are among the places where the risk of transmission of the virus is high will direct individuals to prefer healthcare institutions where the procedures are carried out faster.

Among the studies conducted on demand for health services, according to Hotchkiss (1998), the increase in the patient density in healthcare institutions decreases the health service demand of individuals. According to Lindelow (2005) and Şenol et al. (2010) proximity to the healthcare institution increases individuals' health service demand. As a result of individuals' demand for health services, the shorter time spent in the healthcare institution and the faster execution of procedures increase the demand for private healthcare institutions (Al-Ghanim, 2004; Hanson et al., 2004). These results regarding the demand for healthcare services are in line with the factors affecting the healthcare institution choices of individuals during the COVID-19 pandemic.

Another factor that impacts the healthcare institution choices of the participants during the COVID-19 pandemic is the "Greater scope of services offered." According to Şantaş et al. (2016), healthcare institutions' service scope affects the demand for health services. Another factor affecting the demand for healthcare services is the hygiene and cleanliness of an institution (Sahn et al., 2003; Şantaş et al., 2016). Especially during the COVID-19 pandemic, one of the most important factors affecting individuals' healthcare institution choice is the hygiene and cleanliness status of an institution. Individuals prefer health-care institutions that they perceive as safe in terms of hygiene and cleanliness.

The effect of income status on the participants' healthcare institution choices during the COVID-19 pandemic is evidentiary. During the pandemic, the high-income group participants' healthcare institution preference is "Private hospital/ private medical center," while the participants with low income prefer the "Family health center," which offers free health care. In their studies, Habtom and Ruys (2007) and Saraçoğlu and Öztürk (2016) stated that the increase in the income level increases the demand for "Private hospital/ private medical center" in healthcare institution preferences. These results regarding the demand for healthcare services are in line with the factors affecting the healthcare institution choices of individuals during the COVID-19 pandemic.

As a result, this study fills an important gap in the literature by providing information about the healthcare institution preferences of individuals during a pandemic. This study is thought to become an important guide (source) for the measures to be taken in the fight against the COVID-19 pandemic and other pandemics globally for healthcare managers and politicians.

References

Al-Ghanim, S. A. (2004). Factors influencing the utilisation of public and private primary health care services in Riyadh City. Journal of King Abdulaziz University, 19(1), 3–27. https://www.kau.edu.sa/Files/320/Researches/51714_21849.pdf.

Ateş, M. (2011). Sağlık hizmetleri yönetimi. Beta Yayınları, 2. Baskı.

Aydın, S. (2008). Hayata yüksekten bakabilmek sağlık politikası üzerine makale ve denemeler. Medipolitan Eğitim ve Sağlık Vakfı Yayınları.

Chen, L., Xiong, J., Bao, L., & Shi, Y. (2020). Convalescent plasma as a potential therapy for COVID-19. The Lancet, 20(4), 398–400. https://doi.org/10.1016/S1473-3099(20)30141-9

Çelik, Y. (2019). Sağlık ekonomisi. Siyasal Kitapevi, 4. Baskı.

Family Medicine Law. (2004). Official Newspaper Date: 09.12.2004, No: 25665. Law number: 5258.

Fanelli, D. & Piazza, F. (2020). Analysis and forecast of COVID-19 spreading in China, Italy and France. Chaos, Solitons and Fractals, 134, 1–5. https://doi.org/10.1016/j.chaos.2020.109761

Gorbalenya, A. E., Baker, S. C., Baric, R. S. et al. (2020). The species severe acute respiratory syndrome-related coronavirus: Classifying 2019-nCoV and naming it SARS-CoV-2. Nature Microbiology, 5, 536–544. https://doi. org/10.1038/s41564-020-0695-z

Gu, J., Han, B., & Wang, J. (2020). COVID-19: Gastrointestinal manifestations and potential fecal- oral transmission. Gastroenterology, 158(6), 1518–1519. https://doi.org/10.1053/j.gastro.2020.02.054

Habtom, G. K. & Ruys, P. (2007). The choice of a health care provider in Eritrea. Health Policy, 80(1), 202–217. https://doi.org/10.1016/j.healthpol.2006.02.012

Hanson, K., Yip, W. C., & Hsiao, W. (2004). The impact of quality on the demand for outpatient services in Cyprus. Health Economics, 13(12), 1167–1180. https://doi.org/10.1002/hec.898

Hotchkiss, D. R. (1998). The tradeoff between price and quality of services in the Philippines. Social Science and Medicine, 46(2), 227–242. https://doi. org/10.1016/S0277-9536(97)00152-4

Inpatient Treatment Institutions Management Regulation. (1983). Official Newspaper Date: 13.1.1983, No: 17927.

Kamps, B. S. & Hoffmann, C. (2020). COVID reference. Eng, 4. Edition. https:// amedeo.com/CovidReference04.pdf.

Kavuncubaşı, Ş. & Yıldırım, S. (2015). Hastane ve sağlık kurumları yönetimi. Siyasal Kitabevi, 4. Baskı.

Kılıç, D. & Çalışkan, Z. (2013). Sağlık hizmetleri kullanımı ve davranışsal model. Nevşehir Hacı Bektaş Veli Üniversitesi SBE Dergisi, 2(2), 192–206.

Lai, M. M. C. & Cavanagh, D. (1997). The molecular biology of coronaviruses. Advances in Virus Research, 48, 1–100. http://dx.doi.org/10.1016/ S0065-3527(08)60286-9

Lai, S., Ruktanoncchai, N. W., Zhou, L., Prosper, O., Luo, W., Floyd, J. R., Wesolowski, A. et al. (2020). Effect of non-pharmaceutical interventions to contain COVID-19 in China. Nature 2020; [Epub ahead of print]. https://doi. org/10.1038/s41586-020-2293-x

Lindelow, M. (2005). The utilisation of curative healthcare in Mozambique: Does income matter?. Journal of African Economies, 14(3), 435–482. https://doi. org/10.1093/jae/eji015

Mills, A. & Gilson, L. (1988). Health economics for developing countries: A survival kit. Health Economics & Financing Programme Working Paper Series, No:01/88. http://cphs.huph.edu.vn/uploads/tainguyen/sachvabaocao/ First_Modiriat2.pdf.

Ministry of Health of Turkey. (2018). Sağlık İstatistikleri Yıllığı 2018. T.C. Sağlık Bakanlığı Sağlık Bilgi Sistemleri Genel Müdürlüğü. https://dosyasb. saglik.gov.tr/Eklenti/36134,siy2018trpdf.pdf?0, Access date: 29.07.2020.

Ministry of Health of Turkey. (2019). Sağlık hizmeti sunucularının basamaklandırılması. Sağlık Hizmetleri Genel Müdürlüğü, 31/05/2019 tarihli ve 3274 sayılı Genelge.

Ministry of Health of Turkey. (2020a). 2019-nCoV hastalığı sağlık çalışanları rehberi. Bilim kurulu çalışması. https://hsgm.saglik.gov.tr/depo/haberler/ ncov/2019-nCov_Hastal_Salk_alanlar_Rehberi.pdf.

Ministry of Health of Turkey. (2020b). COVID-19 (SARS-CoV-2 enfeksiyonu) genel bilgiler, epidemiyoloji ve tanı. Bilimsel danışma kurulu çalışması. https://covid19bilgi.saglik.gov.tr/depo/rehberler/covid-19-rehberi/COVID-19_REHBERI_GENEL_BILGILER_EPIDEMIYOLOJI_VE_TANI.pdf.

Mooney, G. (2003). Economics, medicine and health care. England: Pearson Education Limited, 3. Edition.

Murthy, S., Gomersall, C. D., & Fowler, R. A. (2020). Care for critically ill patients with COVID-19. JAMA, 323(15), 1499–1500. https://doi.org/10.1001/ jama.2020.3633

Myint, S. H. (1995). Human coronavirus infections. In: The coronaviridae. Editor: Siddell, S. G., New York, N.Y: Plenum Publishing, 389–401. https:// doi.org/10.1007/978-1-4899-1531-3

Nacoti, M., Ciocca, A., Giupponi, A., Brambillasca, P., Lussana, F. et al. (2020). At the epicenter of the Covid-19 pandemic and humanitarian crises in Italy: Changing perspectives on preparation and mitigation. Innovations in Care Delivery. https://doi.org/10.1056/CAT.20.0080

Naldöken, Ü., Biçer, E. B., & Tosun, N. (2018). Sağlık politikalarında ihtiyaç ve talep, (Ed. Tengilimoğlu, D.), Sağlık Politikası. Nobel Akademik Yayıncılık. 125–136.

Olesen, F. & Fleming, D. (1998). Patient registration and controlled access to secondary care prerequisites for integrated care. European Journal of General Practice, 4(2), 81–83. https://doi.org/10.3109/13814789809160800

Sabino-Silva, R., Jardim, A. C. G., & Siqueira, W. L. (2020). Coronavirus COVID-19 impacts to dentistry and potential salivary diagnosis. Clinical Oral Investigations, 24, 1619–1621. https://doi.org/10.1007/s00784-020-03248-x

Sahn, D. E., Younger, S. D., & Genicot, G. (2003). The demand for health care services in rural Tanzania. Oxford Bulletin of Economics and Statistics, 65(2), 241–260. https://doi.org/10.1111/1468-0084.t01-2-00046

Saraçoğlu, S. & Öztürk, F. (2016). Sağlık hizmetlerine yönelik talebin belirleyicileri: Türkiye üzerine bir uygulama. İş ve Hayat, 2(4), 293–342.

Shaw, R., Kim, Y., & Hua, J. (2020). Governance, technology and citizen behavior in pandemic: Lessons from COVID-19 in East Asia. Progress in Disaster Science, 6, 1–11. https://doi.org/10.1016/j.pdisas.2020.100090

Siddell, S. G. (1995). The coronaviridae. In: The coronaviridae. Editor: Siddell, S. G., New York, NY: Plenum Publishing, 1–10. https://doi.org/10.1007/978-1-4899-1531-3

Şantaş, F., Kurşun, A., & Kar, A. (2016). Hastane tercihine etki eden faktörler: Sağlık hizmetleri pazarlaması perspektifinden alan araştırması. Hacettepe Sağlık İdaresi Dergisi, 19(1), 17–33.

Şenol, V., Çetinkaya, F., & Balcı, E. (2010). Factors associated with health services utilization by the general population in the center of Kayseri, Turkey. Türkiye Klinikleri Tıp Bilimleri Dergisi, 30(2), 721–730. https://doi.org/10.5336/medsci.2008-9283

Tengilimoğlu, D., Işık, O., & Akbolat, M. (2017). Sağlık işletmeleri yönetimi. Nobel Akademik Yayıncılık, 8. Basım.

Tillu, G., Chaturvedi, S., Chopra, A., & Patwardhan, B. (2020). Public health approach of ayurveda and yoga for COVID-19 prophylaxis. The Journal of Alternative and Complementary Medicine, 26(5), 360–364. http://doi.org/10.1089/acm.2020.0129

Turkish Statistical Institute. (2019). Nüfus istatistikleri. http://www.tuik.gov.tr/UstMenu.do?metod=temelist.

Uysal, B. & Ulusinan, E. (2020). The importance of halotherapy in the treatment of COVID-19 related diseases. Journal of Clinical and Experimental Investigations, 11(4), 1–7. https://doi.org/10.29333/jcei/8486

Weiss, R. S. & Leibowitz, J. L. (2011). Coronavirus pathogenesis. Advances in Virus Research, 81, 85–164. http://dx.doi.org/10.1016/B978-0-12-385885-6.00009-2

Weiss, R. S. & Navas- Martin, S. (2005). Coronavirus pathogenesis and the emerging pathogen severe acute respiratory syndrome coronavirus. Microbiology and Molecular Biology Reviews, 69(4), 635–664. http://dx.doi.org/10.1128/MMBR.69.4.635-664.2005

World Health Organization. (2003). Summary table of SARS cases by country, 1 November 2002–7 August 2003. https://www.who.int/csr/sars/country/2003_08_15/en/.

World Health Organization. (2020a). Novel coronavirus (2019-nCoV) situation report-1. https://www.who.int/docs/default-source/coronaviruse/situation-reports/20200121-sitrep-1-2019-ncov.pdf?sfvrsn=20a99c10_4.

World Health Organization. (2020b). Novel coronavirus (2019-nCoV) situation report-10. https://www.who.int/docs/default-source/coronaviruse/situation-reports/20200130-sitrep-10-ncov.pdf?sfvrsn=d0b2e480_2.

World Health Organization. (2020c). WHO Director-General's opening remarks at the media briefing on COVID-19, 11 March 2020. https://www.who.int/dg/speeches/detail/who-director-general-s-opening-remarks-at-the-media-briefing-on-covid-19---11-march-2020.

World Health Organization. (2020d). Novel coronavirus (2019-nCoV) situation report-32. https://www.who.int/docs/default-source/coronaviruse/situation-reports/20200221-sitrep-32-covid-19.pdf.

World Health Organization Regional Office for the Eastern Mediterranean. (2019). Mers situation update September 2019. https://applications.emro.who.int/docs/EMROPub-MERS-SEP-2019-EN.pdf?ua=1&ua=1.

Yang, D. & Leibowitz, J. L. (2015). The structure and functions of coronavirus genomic 3' and 5' Ends. Virus Research, 206, 120–133. https://doi.org/10.1016/j.virusres.2015.02.025

Yaylalı, M., Kaynak, S., & Karaca, Z. (2012). Health services demand: A study in Erzurum. Ege Academic Review, 12(4), 563–573.

Yazıcıoğlu, Y. & Erdoğan, S. (2004). SPSS uygulamalı bilimsel araştırma yöntemleri. Detay Yayıncılık.

Res. Asst. Ebrar Ulusinan

Relationship between Air Pollution and the COVID-19

1. Introduction

Air pollution consists of pollutants caused by both natural resources and humans (anthropogenic) (Genc et al., 2012: 1; Lim et al., 2012: 2226; Kurt et al., 2016: 2). It is defined as the level of pollutants such as lead, carbon monoxide (CO), ozone (O3) (Kurt et al., 2016: 2), sulfur dioxide (SO2), particulate matter (PM) and nitrogen oxide (NOx) in the air we breathe, causing unfavorable effects on the environment and human health (Bayram et al., 2006: 106). Coarse particulate matter (PM10) diameters range from 2.5 to 10 μm, while fine particulate matter (PM 2.5) diameters are less than 2.5 μm (Marcazzan et al., 2001; Pozzi et al., 2003; Xing, 2016). Exposure to fine particles in the environment causes various diseases such as lung cancer(Huang et al., 2017), cardiovascular diseases (Brook et al., 2010), respiratory tract infections, chronic obstructive pulmonary disease and significant health consequences resulting in untimely death (Apte et al., 2018). In this study, PM2.5 particulate matter was considered as air pollution data and analyzes were made on the average annual exposure of this particulate matter.

In other words, air pollution is foreign substances in the atmosphere in the amount and duration that will affect human health and activities, the health and activities of other living things, their belongings and aesthetic dimensions (Bayat, 2011: 56). With the pace of urbanization and the accompanying rise in power consumption, transport and the use of industrial resources, people are exposed not only to more air pollution but also to a more varied range of air pollution (Kelly and Fussell, 2011: 1059).

Although the air pollution level, which has been regularly monitored and struggled for the last 30 years in the world, is still above the safe limits, especially in big cities. This pollution level disrupts the natural balance in the atmosphere and negatively affects public health (Bayram et al., 2006: 106). As a matter of fact, there are many studies proving that air pollution poses a health threat (Samet et al., 2000; Chen et al., 2004; Finkelstein et al., 2004; Dominici et al., 2006; Ciencewicki ve Jaspers, 2007; Qiu et al., 2012; Song et al., 2014; DeVries et al., 2017; Horne et al., 2018; Xie et al., 2019). While air pollution was once thought of as a regional and local problem, it is now addressed as an international problem. Nine out of ten people living in urban areas worldwide have to live with incur air pollution. Decreased lung function is linked to increased airway reactivity in children with asthma. At the same time, prolonged exposure to air pollution raises the risk of asthma in children. Short-term air pollution is one reason for respiratory tract infection symptoms and increased visits to the emergency room (Kurt et al., 2016: 10). With the increase in air pollution, the risk of respiratory diseases such as respiratory infections, asthma and COPD in children and adults increases (Kim et al., 2018: 89). In this context, it can be said that clean air is one of the basic elements of quality of life (Craig et al., 2008: 589).

The COVID-19 pandemic that emerged in Wuhan, one of China's provinces in December 2019 and then spread all over the world, posed a serious threat to human health (Bontempi, 2020: 1; Contini and Costabile, 2020: 1), was caused widespread panic all over the world by posing a serious threat to human health (Zhang et al., 2020: 1). It is thought that the increase and mortality rate of COVID-19 depends on many factors, and one of these factors is air pollution (Uysal et al., 2020). As a matter of fact, it is clear that there are significant distinctions in the spread and mortality rate of the COVID-19 pandemic in world different countries, even in diverse parts of the same country (Contini and Costabile, 2020: 1; Conticini et al., 2020: 1; Frontera et al., 2020). Although there are few comments on the disclosure of the data, it is thought that exposure to air pollutants reduces the population's resistance to COVID-19 and more research is needed (Contini and Costabile, 2020).

The COVID-19 is a respiratory disease and is spread by airborne contamination via aerosols (van Doremalen et al., 2020). Aerosols are "small droplets" suspended in the air. Infectious droplets of different sizes spread around when infected patients cough, breathe or sneeze (Tellier et al., 2019: 2). Under normal conditions, large droplets that spread are stopped in a short time by the resistance of the air and are generally removed at a distance of less than 1–1.5 m from infected person. However, virus-laden particles of an infected patient can stay in the air for a long time and be transmitted by wind. For these reasons, it is predicted that air pollution may facilitate transmission of the disease (Contini and Costabile, 2020: 2).

The COVID-19 pandemic has similarities to the severe acute respiratory syndrome (SARS) caused by SARS-CoV, which emerged in Guangzhou, China in 2003 (Comunian et al., 2020: 3; Wang et al., 2020: L416). SARS deaths varied across geographic regions, similar to COVID-19. Air pollution was predicted to be one of the factors responsible for these changes. As a matter of fact, a study carried out in China showed that exposure to some air pollutants can be dangerous for lung functions and thus increase SARS deaths (Cui et al., 2003).

Many studies have revealed the relationship of air pollution to COVID-19 spread and mortality rates. The study focusing on 120 cities in China is one of them (Zhu et al., 2020). Similarly, a study conducted in 219 cities in China concluded that air pollution indexes were positively associated with newly approved patients (Zhang et al., 2020). Similar results have been obtained in studies examining its contribution of the COVID-19 spread and to mortality rates of pollution concentrations in Italy (Fattorini and Regoli, 2020; Setti et al., 2020). Coccia (2020) conducted a study based on the 7 April 2020 cases and focusing on 55 Italian cities. In this study, it was found that there were approximately 3600 infected patients in cities exposed to air pollution for more than 100 days, whereas there were 1000 infected patients in cities exposed to less than 100 days of air pollution. Hendryx and Luo (2020), in their study focusing on the United States of America (USA), concluded that air pollution is associated with the prevalence of COVID-19 and death. Cole et al. (2020) examined the data of 355 Dutch municipalities and found a statistically significant positive relationship between air pollution and COVID-19 cases, deaths and hospital admissions. Li et al. (2020) in Wuhan and XiaoGan's study examining the relationship of four environmental pollutants and different variables with COVID-19 in the cities, it was observed that two air pollutants strongly support COVID-19 transmission. Another study examining the impact of air pollutants on the COVID-19 pandemic in California concluded that some environmental pollutants have a significant association with the COVID-19 pandemic in California (Bashir et al., 2020).

As seen in the studies which were made, it can be interpreted that exposure to air pollution may increase susceptibility and have harmful effects on patients affected by COVID-19 (Contini and Costabile, 2020). Indeed, the European Public Health Association (EPHA) (2020) warned that those living in polluted cities are at a higher risk of COVID-19.

In this respect, the study aims to examine the relationship between air pollution and the COVID-19 pandemic with variables such as the rate of cumulative case, cumulative cases per million population, cumulative deaths, and cumulative deaths per million population.

2. Methods

The research was done by considering PM2.5 particulate matterData related to PM2.5 was obtained from the World Bank. Since the most up-to-date data belongs to 2017, this date is based on. The study included 21 countries with average annual exposure (micrograms per cubic meter) of PM2.5 air pollution higher than 50.49 and 57 countries lower than 15.02. Data related to COVID-19 were derived from WHO (13 September 2020) data. The data of cumulative cases, cumulative cases per million population, cumulative deaths, and cumulative deaths per million population were used in the published report. The 21 countries with the highest pollution level and 57 countries with the lowest pollution level were grouped and a comparison analysis was made. Data were analyzed with SPSS 22.0. In addition to descriptive statistics to analyze the data, normality test and Mann-Whitney U test to make comparison between groups were used.

3. Results

Analysis results of the normality test performed to determine the test techniques to be used in the analysis are shown in Tab. 1. Since p <0.05 as a result of the normality test of the data and the distribution did not show a normal distribution, the analysis was performed according to non-parametric test techniques.

Looking at the descriptive statistics of the variables in Tab. 2, it is seen that the maximum pollution level of the countries in the first group is 99.73. The lowest pollution level of the countries in the second group, whose micrograms per cubic meter is less than 15.02, is 5.81.

In 21 countries with the highest pollution level, the minimum number of cases is Chad with 1083 cases. Chad ranks 10th in terms of average annual exposure to PM2.5 air pollution with a rate of 66.02. The country with the maximum number of cases in the first group of countries is India with 4754356 cases. India ranks 4th with 90.87 pollutions. In 57 countries with the lowest pollution levels, there are 8 countries with no cases to date (Marshall Islands, Tonga, Kiribati, Micronesia, Fed. Sts., Samoa, Vanuatu, Solomon Islands,

Tab. 1. Tests of normality

| | Shapiro-Wilk | | |
	Statistic	df	Sig.
PM2.5 pollution	,687	78	,000
Cumulative cases	,269	78	,000
Cumulative cases per million population	,704	78	,000
Cumulative deaths	,310	78	,000
Cumulative deaths per million population	,706	78	,000

Tab. 2. Descriptive statistics of variables

Variables	Country groups according to PM2.5	N	Descriptive Statistics			
			mean	sd	min	max
PM2.5 pollution	>50,49	21	69,21	16,00	50,49	99,73
	<15,02	57	10,71	2,51	5,81	15,02
Cumulative cases	>50,49	21	318628	1022689	1083	4754356
	<15,02	57	247912	1006054	0	6386832
Cumulative cases per million population	>50,49	21	6641	11761	49	42180
	<15,02	57	5126	5883	0	23253
Cumulative deaths	>50,49	21	5620	16904	62	78586
	<15,02	57	8921	30894	0	191809
Cumulative deaths per million population	>50,49	21	51	52	3	197
	<15,02	57	175	227	0	856

(**Note**: The expressions that are <1 in Cumulative cases per million population and Cumulative deaths per million population data have been changed to 0 for analysis.)

American Samoa). The country with the maximum number of cases in the second group of countries is the United States with 6386832 cases. The United States of America is the 186th country with 7.40 in the average annual exposure to PM2.5 air pollution.

Considering the cumulative case data per million population of country groupings, the lowest country in countries with an average annual exposure of over 50.49 to air pollution is Niger with 49 cases. Niger ranks 2nd in pollution with a rate of 94.05. The maximum case is Qatar with 42180 cases. Qatar is the third country with 91.18 pollutions. In countries with average annual exposure to air pollution less than 15.02, the country with the highest cumulative number of cases per million population is Panama. Panama is the 165th country with 11.40 pollution.

Looking at the cumulative death data of country groupings, the Central African Republic is the minimum case with 62 cases in countries with an average annual exposure of over 50.49 to air pollution. The Central African Republic is the 16th country with 56.82 pollutions. The maximum case is India with 78586 cases. In countries with an average annual exposure of less than 15.02 to air pollution, the country with the highest cumulative deaths is the United States with 191809 cases.

Considering the cumulative death data per million population of country groupings, the lowest country in the countries in the first group is Niger with 3

Tab. 3. Comparison of country groups according to PM2.5 (Source: The World Bank, 2017)

Variables	Country groups according to PM2.5	N	p
Cumulative Cases	>50,49	21	,021*
	<15,02	57	
Cumulative cases per million population	>50,49	21	,809
	<15,02	57	
Cumulative deaths	>50,49	21	,065
	<15,02	57	
Cumulative deaths per million population	>50,49	21	,225
	<,15,02	57	

deaths. The maximum death is Iraq with 197 cases. Iraq ranks 11th with 61.63 pollutions. In countries with average annual exposure to air pollution less than 15.02, the country with the highest cumulative deaths per million population is Belgium with 856 cases. Belgium is the 148th country with 12.88 pollutions.

The Mann-Whitney U test was conducted to compare 21 countries with the highest pollution level and 57 countries with the lowest pollution level. According to the analysis, there is a statistically significant difference between country groupings in terms of cumulative case scores ($p < 0.05$). Accordingly, cumulative deaths differ according to the average annual exposure of countries to PM2.5 air pollution. Cumulative case rates appear to be higher in countries with average annual exposure to PM2.5 air pollution> 50.49.

According to the other results of the analysis, no statistically significant difference was found between country groups and Cumulative cases per million population, Cumulative deaths and Cumulative deaths per million population data according to PM2,5.

When the average annual exposure of the countries to PM2.5 air pollution is examined in Fig. 1, Finland is the country with the lowest pollution level. Brunei Darussalam and New Zealand follow Finland. Haiti is the country with the highest pollution level in this group with 15.01 pollution.

Looking at the average annual exposure of countries to PM2.5 air pollution in Fig. 2, Nepal is the country with the highest pollution level with 99.73 pollution. Niger and Qatar follow Nepal. Uganda is the country with the lowest pollution level in this group with 50.49 pollution.

Considering the figure above, the density of countries according to their annual average exposure to PM2.5 air pollution is seen.

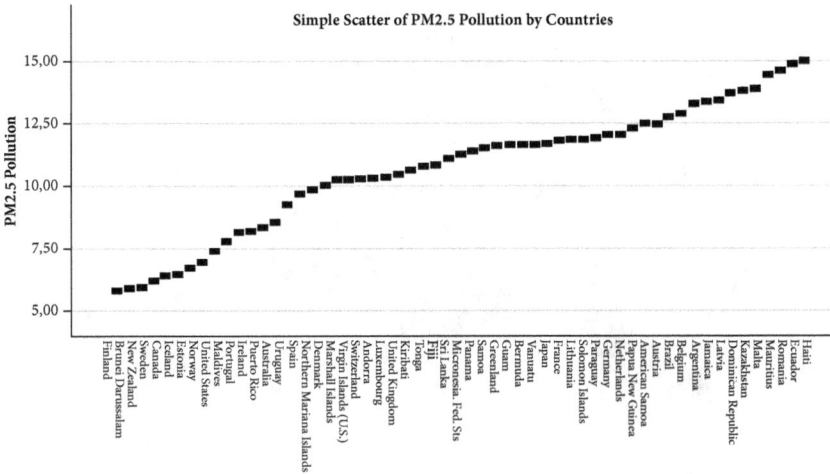

Fig. 1. 57 countries with average annual exposure (micrograms per cubic meter) to PM2.5 air pollution lower than 15.02 (Source: The World Bank, 2017)

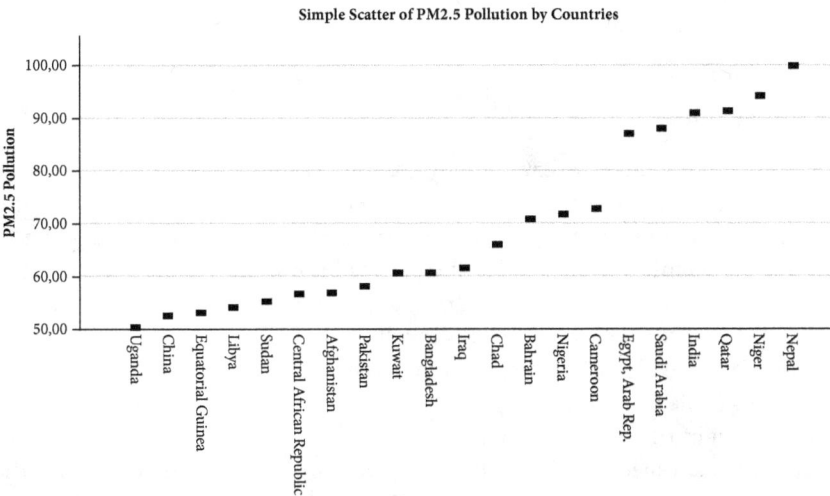

Fig. 2. 21 countries with average annual exposure (micrograms per cubic meter) to PM2.5 air pollution above 50.49 (Source: The World Bank, 2017)

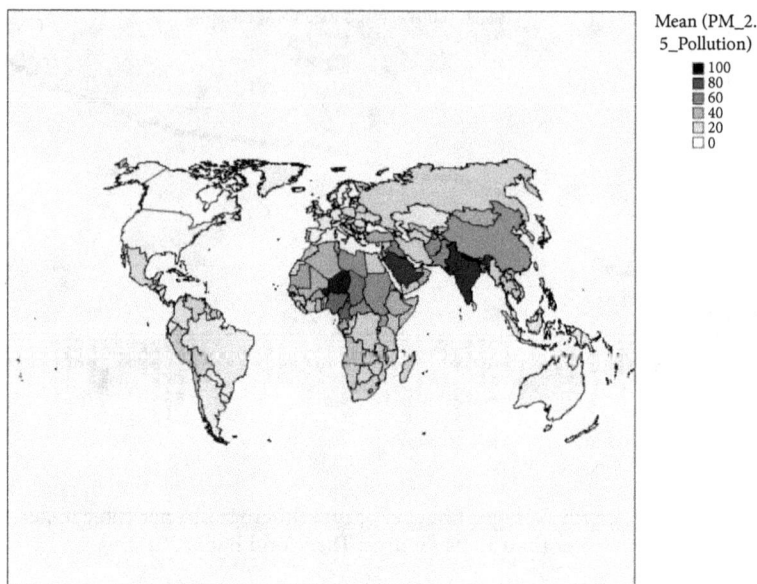

Fig. 3. World map by average annual exposure of countries to PM2.5 air pollution (Source: The World Bank, 2017)

4. Discussion

For nearly nine months, every country has been trying to take measures per its economic structure to control the COVID-19 pandemic, which the entire world has been struggling with. Governments and health systems are struggling to contain isolate millions of people, the spread of the virus and prevent hospitals from facing extreme congestion. To counter this unprecedented pandemic, it is important for policymakers and healthcare professionals to know which groups are at greater risk of disease and death, and which factors may increase these risks (Cole et al., 2020).

It is thought that air pollution, which has significant damages to the health of individuals, especially respiratory systems, is one factors that increase the risk of exposure and the severity of the disease. As a result of this study based on this idea, some important data were got. No COVID-19 cases have been observed so far in 8 of the 57 countries with average annual exposure of less than 15.02 to air pollution. In 21 countries with the highest pollution level, there is no country with no cases, but the lowest number of cases is Chad with

1083 cases. According to the Mann-Whitney U test conducted between the two country groups, cumulative measurements differed according to the average annual exposure of the countries to PM2.5 air pollution. In this context, it can be said that countries with an average annual exposure to PM2.5 air pollution> 50.49 will have higher cumulative cases. This is like many studies examining the relationship between air pollution and COVID-19 (Coker et al., 2020; Frontera et al., 2020; Hou et al., 2020).

Although it is known that the COVID-19 pandemic differs according to many variables, the importance of air pollution should not be ignored. As a matter of fact, exposure to air pollution poses not only a danger during the COVID-19 pandemic process. Breathing clean air is a basic need for our health in all conditions. In this context, it is necessary to make local and global efforts to ensure better breathing air. As for the COVID-19 pandemic process, focusing on the vulnerable population exposed to long-term air pollution can be helpful (Hou et al., 2020).

As a result, as emphasized in many studies, individuals in countries exposed to air pollution are considered to be at a disadvantage during the COVID-19 process. Therefore, it is important that governments and private companies make regulations on the subject.

References

Apte, J. S., Brauer, M., Cohen, A. J. et al. (2018). Ambient PM2.5 reduces global and regional life expectancy. Environmental Science & Technology Letters, 5(9), 546–551. https://doi.org/10.1021/acs.estlett.8b00360

Bashir, M. F., MA, M. J., Komal, B. et al. (2020). Correlation between environmental pollution indicators and COVID-19 pandemic: A brief study in Californian context. Environmental Research, 187, 109652, https://doi.org/10.1016/j.envres.2020.109652

Bayat, B. (2011). Hava Kirliliği ve Kontrolü. Bilim ve Aklın Aydınlığında Eğitim, 135, 55–59.

Bayram, H., Dörtbudak, Z., Evyapan Fişekçi, F., Kargın, M., & Bülbül, B. (2006). Hava Kirliliğinin İnsan Sağlığına Etkileri, Dünyada, Ülkemizde ve Bölgemizde Hava Kirliliği Sorunu. Paneli Ardından. Dicle Tıp Dergisi, 33(2), 105–112.

Bontempi, E. (2020). Commercial exchanges instead of air pollution as possible origin of COVID19 initial diffusion phase in Italy: More efforts are necessary to address interdisciplinary research. Environmental Research, 188, 109775. https://doi.org/10.1016/j.envres.2020.109775

Chen, B., Hong, C., & Kan, H. (2004). Exposures and health outcomes from outdoor air pollutants in China. Toxicology, 198, 291–300. doi: 10.1016/j.tox.2004.02.005

Ciencewicki, J. & Jaspers, I. (2007). Air pollution and respiratory viral infection. Inhalation Toxicology, 19(14), 1135–1146. doi: 10.1080/08958370701665434

Coccia, M. (2020). Factors determining the diffusion of COVID-19 and suggested strategy to prevent future accelerated viral infectivity similar to COVID. Science of the Total Environment, 729. https://doi.org/10.1016/j.scitotenv.2020.138474.

Cohen, J. & Normile, D. (2020). New SARS-like virus in China triggers alarm. Science, 367(6475), 234–235, doi: 10.1126/science.367.6475.234

Coker, E. S., Cavalli, L., Fabrizi, E. et al. (2020). The effects of air pollution on COVID-19 related mortality in Northern Italy. Environmental and Resource Economics. https://doi.org/10.1007/s10640-020-00486-1

Cole, M. A., Ozgen, C., & Strobl, E. (2020). Air pollution exposure and Covid-19 in Dutch municipalities. Environmental and Resource Economics. https://doi.org/10.1007/s10640-020-00491-4

Comunian, S., Dongo, D., Milani, C., & Palestini, P. (2020). Air pollution and COVID-19: The role of particulate matter in the spread and increase of COVID-19's morbidity and mortality. International Journal of Environmental Research and Public Health, 17(12), 4487; https://doi.org/10.3390/ijerph17124487.

Conticini, E., Frediani, B., & Caro, D. (2020). Can atmospheric pollution be considered a co-factor in extremely high level of SARS-CoV-2 lethality in Northern Italy? Environmental Pollution, 261, 114465, https://doi.org/10.1016/j.envpol.2020.114465

Contini, D. & Costabile, F. (2020). Does air pollution influence COVID-19 outbreaks?. Atmosphere, 11(4), 377. https://doi.org/10.3390/atmos11040377

Craig, L., Brook, J. R., Chiotti, Q. et al. (2008). Air pollution and public health: A guidance document for risk managers. Journal of Toxicology and Environmental Health, Part A, 71, 9–10, 588–698. doi: 10.1080/15287390801997732

Cui, Y., Zhang, Z., Froines, J. et al. (2003). Air pollution and case fatality of SARS in the People's Republic of China: An ecologic study. Environmental Health, 2(15). https://doi.org/10.1186/1476-069X-2-15

DeVries, R., Kriebel, D., & Sama, S. (2017). Outdoor air pollution and COPD-related emergency department visits, hospital admissions, and mortality: A meta-analysis. COPD: Journal of Chronic Obstructive Pulmonary Disease, 14(1), 113–121. https://doi.org/10.1080/15412555.2016.1216956

Dominici, F., Peng, R. D., Bell, M. L. et al. (2006). Fine Particulate Air Pollution and Hospital Admission for Cardiovascular and Respiratory Diseases. JAMA, 295(10), 1127–34.

European Public Health Alliance. (Mar 16, 2020). Coronavirus threat greater for polluted cities2, https://epha.org/coronavirus-threat-greater-for-polluted-cities/, Access date: 09.11.2020.

Fattorini, D. & Regoli, F. (2020). Role of the chronic air pollution levels in the Covid-19 outbreak risk in Italy. Environmental Pollution, 264. https://doi.org/10.1016/j.envpol.2020.114732

Finkelstein, M. M., Jerrett, M., & Sears, M. R. (2004). Traffic air pollution and mortality rate advancement periods. American Journal of Epidemiology, 160(2), 173–177. https://doi.org/ 10.1093 / aje / kwh181

Frontera, A., Cianfanelli, L., Vlachos, K. et al. (2020). Severe air pollution links to higher mortality in COVID-19 patients: The "double-hit" hypothesis. Journal of Infection, 81(2), 255–259. https://doi.org/10.1016/j.jinf.2020.05.031

Genc, S., Zadeoglulari, Z., Fuss, S. H., & Genc, K. (2012). The adverse effects of air pollution on the nervous system. Journal of Toxicology, doi: 10.1155/2012/782462

Hendryx, M. & Luo, J. (2020). COVID-19 prevalence and fatality rates in association with air pollution emission concentrations and emission sources. Environmental Pollution, 265, 115126. https://doi.org/10.1016/j.envpol.2020.115126

Horne, B. D., Joy, E. A., Hofmann, M. G. et al. (2018). Short-term elevation of fine particulate matter air pollution and acute lower respiratory infection. American Journal of Respiratory and Critical Care Medicine, 198, 759–766. https://doi.org/10.1164/rccm.201709-1883OC

Hou, C., Qin, Y., Liu, Q., Yang, X., & Wang, H. (2020). Impact of long-term air pollution on the case fatality rate of COVID-19. Research Square. https://doi.org/10.21203/rs.3.rs-42283/v1

Huang, F., Pan, B., Wu, J., Chen, E., & Chen, L. (2017). Relationship between exposure to PM2.5 and lung cancer incidence and mortality: A meta-analysis. Oncotarget, 8(26), 43322–43331. https://doi.org/10.18632/oncotarget.17313

Kelly, F. J. & Fussell, J. C. (2011). Air pollution and airway disease. Clinical & Experimental Allergy, 41, 1059–1071. doi: 10.1111/j.1365-2222.2011.03776.x

Kim, D., Chen, Z., Zhou, L. F., & Huang, S. X. (2018). Air pollutants and early origins of respiratory diseases. Chronic Diseases and Translational Medicine, 4(2), 75–94. https://doi.org/10.1016/j.cdtm.2018.03.003

Kurt, O. K., Zhang, J., & Pinkerton, K. E. (2016). Pulmonary health effects of air pollution. Current opinion in pulmonary medicine, 22(2), 138–143. https://doi.org/10.1097/MCP.0000000000000248

Li, H., Xu, X. L., Dai, D. W. et al. (2020). Air pollution and temperature are associated with increased COVID-19 incidence: A time series study. International Journal of Infectious Diseases, 97, 278–282. https://doi.org/10.1016/j.ijid.2020.05.076

Lim, S. S., Vos, T., Flaxman, A. D. et al. (2012). A comparative risk assessment of burden of disease and injury attributable to 67 risk factors and risk factor clusters in 21 regions, 1990–2010: A systematic analysis for the Global Burden of Disease Study 2010. The Lancet, 380, 2224–2260. https://doi.org/10.1016/S0140-6736(12)61766-8

Marcazzan, G. M., Vaccaro, S., Valli, G., & Vecchi, R. (2001). Characterisation of PM10 and PM2.5 particulate matter in the ambient air of Milan (Italy). Atmospheric Environment, 35(27), 4639–4650. https://doi.org/10.1016/S1352-2310(01)00124-8

Pozzi, R., De Berardis, B., Paoletti, L., & Guastadisegni, C. (2003). Inflammatory mediators induced by coarse (PM2.5–10) and fine (PM2.5) urban air particles in RAW 264.7 cells. Toxicology, 183(1–3), 243–254. https://doi.org/10.1016/S0300-483X(02)00545-0

Qiu, H., Tak-sun Yu, I., Tian, L. et al. (2012). Effects of coarse particulate matter on emergency hospital admissions for respiratory diseases: A time-series analysis in Hong Kong. Environmental Health Perspectives, 120(4), 572–576.

Samet, J. M., Dominici, F., Curriero, F. C. et al. (2000) Fine particulate air pollution and mortality in 20US Cities, 1987–1994. The New England Journal of Medicine, 343(24), 1742–1749. https://doi.org/10.1056/nejm200012143432401

Setti, L., Passarini, F., de Gennaro, G. et al. (2020). Evaluation of the potential relationship between Particulate Matter (PM) pollution and COVID-19 infection spread in Italy. SIMA Position Paper. http://www.simaonlus.it/wpsima/wp-content/uploads/2020/03/COVID_19_position-paper_ENG.pdf, Access date: 09.11.2020.

Song, Q., Christiani, D. C., Wang, X. et al. (2014). The global contribution of outdoor air pollution to the incidence, prevalence, mortality and hospital admission for chronic obstructive pulmonary disease: A systematic review and meta-analysis. International Journal of Environmental Research and Public Health, 11, 11822–11832. doi:10.3390/ijerph111111822

Tellier, R., Li, Y., Cowling, B. J. et al. (2019). Recognition of aerosol transmission of infectious agents: A commentary. BMC Infectious Diseases, 19, 101. https://doi.org/10.1186/s12879-019-3707-y

The World Bank. (2017). PM2.5 air pollution, mean annual exposure (micrograms per cubic meter). https://data.worldbank.org/indicator/EN.ATM.PM25.MC.M3?end=2017&most_recent_value_desc=true&start=2017&type=shaded&view=map&year=2017 (AD: 18.09.2020).

Uysal, B., Demirkıran, M., & Yorulmaz, M. (2020). Assessing of factors effecting COVID-19 mortality rate on a global basis. Turkish Studies, 15(4), 1185–1192. https://dx.doi.org/10.7827/TurkishStudies.44390

van Doremalen, N., Bushmaker, T., Morris, D. H. et al. (2020). Aerosol and surface stability of SARS-CoV-2 as compared with SARS-CoV-1. N. Engl. J. Med., 382, 1564–1567. https://doi.org/10.1056/NEJMc2004973.

Wang, B., Chen, H., Chan, Y. L. & Oliver, B. G. (2020). Is there an association between the level of ambient air pollution and COVID-19?. American Journal of Physiology-Lung Cellular and Molecular Physiology, 319, L416–L421. doi:10.1152/ajplung.00244.2020

World Health Organization. (2020). Coronavirus disease (COVID-19) Weekly Epidemiological Update. https://www.who.int/docs/default-source/coronaviruse/situation-reports/20200914-weekly-epi-update-5.pdf?sfvrsn=cf929d04_2, Access date: 08.11.2020.

Xie, J., Teng, J., Fan, Y. et al. (2019). The short-term effects of air pollutants on hospitalizations for respiratory disease in Hefei, China. International Journal of Biometeorology, 63, 315–326. https://doi.org/10.1007/s00484-018-01665-y

Xing, Y. F., Xu, Y. H., Shi, M. H., & Lian, Y. X. (2016). The impact of PM2.5 on the human respiratory system. Journal of Thoracic Disease, 8(1), E69–E74. https://doi.org/10.3978/j.issn.2072-1439.2016.01.19

Zhang, Z., Xue, T., & Jin, X. (2020). Effects of meteorological conditions and air pollution on COVID-19 transmission: Evidence from 219 Chinese cities. Science of the Total Environment, 741, 140244 https://doi.org/10.1016/j.scitotenv.2020.140244

Zhu, Y., Xie, J., Huang, F., & Cao, L. (2020). Association between short-term exposure to air pollution and COVID-19 infection: Evidence from China. Science of the Total Environment, Elsevier, 727, 138704. https://doi.org/10.1016/j.scitotenv.2020.138704

Asst. Prof. Burhanettin Uysal

Analysis of the Cancellation Reasons of the Tenders Made by Turkish Ministry of Health during the COVID-19 Pandemic

1. Introduction

For individuals to survive or keep their quality of life at a certain level, many types of needs must be met. Even if some endless needs are met, additional needs take their place. However, the limited resources of both society and individuals do not meet unlimited needs. For this reason, both societies and individuals can meet some of their endless needs with limited resources. They try to maximize the level of benefit they will realize while using their limited resources (Çelik, 2016: 99). As Maslow states in the hierarchy of needs (physiological, security, social, respectability, and self-realization), people's needs and desires have priority. According to this order of priority, people strive to meet their needs (Wahba and Bridwell, 1973: 515; Koçel, 2011: 623). For some crucial events that humanity has gone through, the physical and security needs that Maslow has specified separately in the hierarchy of needs can be conjoined. The COVID-19 pandemic is one of the crucial events that confront humanity. And the need for security for people to be protected from the epidemic and to survive can be seen as a kind of physical need.

The COVID-19 (SARS-CoV-2), which emerged in Wuhan, China, in December 2019 (Liu et al., 2020: 1; Lu et al., 2020; Tan et al., 2020: 61; WHO, 2020), caused an international respiratory disease (Cao et al., 2020: 1787). The disease with symptoms such as fever, dry cough, respiratory distress (dyspnea), headache, and pneumonia can cause death with respiratory failure (Zhou et al., 2020). The rapid increase in cases has made the prevention and control of COVID-19 extremely important (Zheng et al., 2020). As a result of the measures taken, essential and unprecedented changes have occurred in society. Because of these changes, the demand for many goods and services has decreased since February (Cicala et al., 2020: 1). Especially personal protective equipment has an essential place among the goods causing this change. This equipment; gloves, face masks, respirators, goggles, face shields, air-purifying respirators, and gowns. This equipment, which was very insignificant before the pandemic, came to the fore with the epidemic and became one of the most preferred equipment. Because of the excessive demand for personal protective equipment, problems that arise in production processes can pose a significant problem in the fight against the epidemic. Because considering that healthcare workers are at the forefront of combating the coronavirus, it is an undeniable fact that they need this equipment the most (Livingston et al., 2020). In this respect, providing personal protective equipment to healthcare workers is a crucial issue in combating the pandemic (Polat and Coşkun, 2020). From this perspective, it is necessary to provide personal protective equipment to health-care workers in a comprehensive, timely, and complete manner under the lead-ership of relevant public institutions and organizations. In these procurement processes, planning nationally is required.

Planning is an administrative method that provides a rational basis for deciding. Choices must be made when demands exceed the resources avail-able, and options must be carefully considered if decisions are to be handled productively and intelligently. Perhaps the most important contribution of pla-nning is the allocation of scarce resources to ensure that health services are made equally available. National health plan comprises the steps of defining the health problems of the society, determining the needs and resources, establishing realistic and applicable targets, and determining the adminis-trative plan needed to achieve the targets (Mejia and Fülöp, 1978: 15–16). The Turkish Ministry of Health has the mandate and authority to take these steps related to national health planning in Turkey. The first policy among these tasks and powers is the protection and development of public health, reducing and preventing disease risks. Another policy is to prevent the entry of public health problems seen in other countries (Turkish Ministry of Health, 2020). Since the COVID-19 Pandemic is also a significant public health problem, the Turkish Ministry of Health has a leading role in the diagnosis, treatment, and reha-bilitation of pandemic-related diseases as well as preventing the entry of sick people into the country and taking necessary precautions.

For people to continue their lives and engage in economic activities, they must protect and maintain their health. However, it has to be spent some money on this. In societies that have brought the level of economic development to a certain level, health awareness increases with the increase in resources allocated for health. While health expenditures play a fundamental role in economic development, they differ according to the development level of the countries. Besides these, it is seen that the share allocated to health expenditures in devel-oped countries is higher than that of developing countries. Health expenditures are variables shaped by the health policies implemented in the country and the sociocultural factors of the country. In other words, health expenditures are accepted as "expenditures for all protection, development, well-being, care, and emergency programs that adopt the aim of protecting and improving health" (Ağır and Tıraş, 2018: 644–646).

Health expenditures are divided into two as current health expenditure and investment expenditure. Among the current health expenditures, hospitals, home nursing care, outpatient care providers, retail sales and other medical supplies, presentation and management of public health programs, general health management, and insurance are other unclassified expenses (TURKSTAT, 2020a). Looking at the statistics of national health expenditures (public and private sector) in 2018, it increased by 17.5 % compared to 2017 and reached 165 billion 234 million Turkish Lira (TL). Approximately 78 % of this belongs to the public sector. The remaining part belongs to the private sector. The ratio of total health expenditure to Gross domestic product (GDP) was 4.4 % in 2018, while the ratio of general government health expenditure to GDP was 3.4 %. While the share of current health expenditure in total health expenditure was 93.1 % in 2017, it became 93.8 % in 2018. The highest number of current health expenditures belongs to hospitals with 52 %. After the expenditures for hospitals, 51.3 % of the expenditures on retail sales and other medical supplies are followed. When we look at the public and private sector expenditures within this expenditure, 76 % of it is the public sector, and 24 % is the private sector. Spending on retail sales and other medical supplies in the government sector increased by 23 % compared to 2017. As seen, the expenditures for retail sales and other medical equipment suppliers in the government sector in 2018 were around 25 % (TURKSTAT, 2020b).

For the government to spend on retail sales and other medical supplies, a procurement transaction must be carried out by the public administrations, and the procurement process must be terminated by accounting for the accrual transaction file. Procurement procedures of public administrations are carried out within the framework of the Public Procurement Legislation. In the legislation, the Public Procurement Law (PPL) No. 4734, the State Procurement Law No. 2886, the Public Procurement Contracts Law No. 4735, the regulations related to the laws, communiques, Public Procurement Board Decisions, etc. are located. Public administrations carry out almost all of their procurement (goods, services, construction work, and consultancy) operations within the framework of the PPL No. 4734, and the public administrations within the PPL are clearly stated in the second article of the PPL. This Law also made a regulation for exception purchases. For example, purchases from the State Supply Office (SSO). Therefore, all purchases are carried out by tenders except for purchases covered by the exception, direct supply purchases, and design contests. In the 18th article of the PPL numbered 4734, the tender procedures to be applied in the procurement of goods or services and construction works (art.19 Open procedure, art.20 restricted procedure, and art. 21 negotiated procedure) are stated. Since the subject of the study is tender, only tenders are mentioned.

In the study, it is aimed to examine the cancellation reasons for the tenders that have a place in public health expenditures. In this direction, information and findings got from the tender statistics presented to the public on the Electronic Public Procurement Platform (EPPP) of the Public Procurement Authority will be presented and some suggestions will be made.

2. Methods

The study is a retrospective study conducted by the descriptive scanning model method. For getting data, the top administration was chosen as the Turkish Ministry of Health in the EPPP database, which is the tender platform of the Public Procurement Authority, according to the Public Procurement Law No. 4734. When selecting the data scanning interval, the start date of the COVID-19 pandemic in Turkey is based on March 11, 2020. Based on the tenders canceled by the administrations affiliated to the Turkish Ministry of Health in the EKAP system between 11.03.2020–31.08.2020. Comparisons were made according to the number of canceled tenders between March 11–August 31, in 2014–2019 years.

SPSS 22.0 program was used in the analysis of the data. For the data that were not normally distributed, non-parametric test techniques were used. The Mann-Whitney U test was used for paired comparisons, and the Kruskal-Wallis H test was used for comparisons in over two groups. The relationship between the dependent and independent variables was analyzed by the Spearman Correlation. I studied it with a 95 % confidence interval and a 5 % margin of error.

3. Results

Looking at the tenders canceled between March 11 and August 31 in 2014–2019; the cancellation average of open procedure goods tenders is 338, the average of open procedure service tenders is 201, and the cancellation average of open procedure construction works tenders is 80. Compared to 2020, the number of cancellations of goods procurement tenders is close to the average of 2014–2019. There is a 12 % decrease in the cancellation status of services tenders, and a 56 % decrease when looking at the cancellation status of the construction works tenders. Accordingly, it is seen that the highest decrease is in the construction works tenders (Tab. 1).

Tab. 1. Procurements canceled for March-August in 2014–2020.

Procurement Type and Procedure	2014		2015		2016		2017		2018		2019		2020	
	n	%	n	%	n	%	n	%	N	%	n	%	n	%
Goods-Open	352	.53	336	.5	298	.52	343	.54	337	.57	359	.59	330	.61
Goods -Negotiated	0	.00	4	.01	0	0	2	0	3	.01	3	0	0	0
Services-Open	202	.31	245	.37	193	.34	185	.29	176	.3	206	.34	176	.32
Services-Negotiated	4	.01	3	0	2	0	1	0	1	0	0	0	0	0
Construction-Open	99	.15	83	.12	79	.14	102	.16	75	.13	43	.07	37	.07
Construction-Negotiated	2	0	0	0	0	0	0	0	0	0	0	0	0	0
Consultancy-Restricted	0	0	0	0	0	0	1	0	0	0	0	0	0	0
Total	659	100	671	100	572	100	634	100	592	100	611	100	543	100

Tab. 2. Type and procedure of canceled procurements and statistical information on partial tender (Source: Public Procurement Authority, 2020)

Procurement Type and Procedure	Partial Tender Type		Total
	Can be given	Cannot be given	
Goods-Open	227	103	330
Services-Open	37	139	176
Construction-Open	7	30	37
Total	271	272	543

Canceled goods purchase procurements with 330 are approximately twice as much as service purchase tenders and 10 times more than construction tenders. On the other hand, all of the canceled procurements are open procedure. There are no tenders canceled by negotiated procedure and restricted procedure. Among the procurements canceled in 2020, there is only 1 procurement with a registration number in 2019.

Considering whether the canceled procurements are open to partial tender, it can be said that they are half-and-half. The status of partial tender in services and construction work procurements is relatively low according to the procurements for the purchase of goods.

Tab. 3. Cross-tabulation of the reason of cancellation with procurement type and procedures (Source: Public Procurement Authority, 2020)

Reasons for Cancellation	Procurement Type and Procedure			Total
	Goods-Open	Services-Open	Construction-Open	
1. The Fact That All Offers Are Well above the Allowance/Approximate Cost for Purchase	48	40	8	96
2. Procurement Commission Decision for e-Evaluation	4	1	1	6
3. Procurement Authority Decision for e-Evaluation	0	0	1	1
4. Not Appropriate Administrative Specifications	3	3	1	7
5. Deficiencies or Errors Regarding the Procurement Announcement	5	6	1	12
6. Changing of the Procurement Procedure	3	2	1	6
7. The Failure of the Tenderer to Sign a Contract	0	1	0	1
8. Change in the Quality or Amount of the Procurement	12	11	0	23
9. No Tenderer with a Valid Tender for the Procurement	50	32	10	92
10. No Tenderer with a Tender for the Procurement	56	34	2	92
11. Noticing the Missing of Procurement Documents Outside the Announcement, Technical, and Administrative Specifications	2	3	2	7
12. Cancellation by Administration upon Complaint	1	1	0	2
13. Cancellation with the Decision of the Public Procurement Board on the Complaint	0	10	0	10
14. Nonconformity of the Technical Specification	12	12	2	26
15. Prohibition / Public Prosecution About the Confirmed Tenderer	0	1	0	1
16. Within the Scope COVID-19 Precautions	8	8	0	16
17. The President's Decree dated 10.06.2020 and numbered 31151/2645	51	0	0	51
18. Administrative Errors and Deficiencies	9	3	6	18
19. Based on the Subject of the SSO Health Market	33	0	0	33
20. Not comply with the Technical Specifications	7	0	0	7
21. No Competition	3	3	0	6
22. For Administrative Reasons	13	2	1	16
23. Other	11	3	1	15
Total	330	176	37	543
Percentage	0.61	0.32	0.07	1.00

The canceled procurement types are goods, services and construction works, all of which are announced by open procedure. There are no procurements for consultancy services, but canceled. On the other hand, there are no tenders that are canceled in the negotiated procedure and restricted procedure. It is seen that the most canceled procurement type among the canceled procurement is the open procedure goods procurement. When the procurement statistics of the Public Procurement Authority (PPA) for the years 2015–2019 are examined, according to the types of public purchases made with PPL No. 4734, the ratio of the purchase of goods procurements in total tenders is in the first place with 41.97 %. Service procurement procurements are second with 35.66 %, construction work procurements are third with 22.10 %, and consultancy procurements are fourth with 0.27 % (Public Procurement Authority, 2020).

When we look at the canceled open goods procurements, it ranks first with a ratio of 61 %. The rate of canceled open procedure services procurements is in the second with 32 %. The rate of canceled open procedure construction works is in third with 0.07 %.

In the list of cancellation reasons for goods procurement with open procedure, the first place is the reason for "No Tenderer with a Tender for the Procurement" with 56 cancellations. Considering this reason, tenders who will participate in the procurement are waited by the administration until the procurement time, and if no tender offer envelope is submitted to the administration, the tender is canceled by the procurement commission because no tenderer has taken part in the procurement. The second among the reasons for canceled procurements is the "President's Decree dated 10.06.2020 and numbered 31151/2645" published in the Official Gazette with 51 cancellations. In this decision, the needs to be met through the SSO have been mentioned. Even if it is advertised, it is obligatory to cancel the procurements by the administrations based on the President's Decree. Administrations may cancel the tender, provided that the reason is shown. This issue has been stated under the heading of "Canceling the procurement before the procurement time" in Article 16 of the PPL No. 4734. The third place among the canceled procurements is the "No Tenderer with a Valid Tender for the Procurement" with 50 cancellations. After the tenderers submit their procurement tender envelopes to the administration, all tender envelopes are opened by the procurement commission. If the tenders are checked, and some cases do not comply with the procurement document and legislation, the tender is deemed invalid. Another vital reason for cancellation is the decision to make the purchase transaction through the SSO. Even if the announcement is made, if the needed goods are available in the SSO,

Tab. 4. Reasons for cancellation of goods procurement (Source: Public Procurement Authority, 2020)

Reasons for Cancellation	Procurement Type and Procedure
	Goods-Open
1. No Tenderer with a Tender for the Procurement	56
2. The President's Decree dated 10.06.2020 and numbered 31151/2645	51
3. No Tenderer with a Valid Tender for the Procurement	50
4. The Fact That All Offers Are Well above the Allowance/Approximate Cost for Purchase	48
5. Based on the Subject of the SSO Health Market	33
6. For Administrative Reasons	13
7. Change in the Quality or Amount of the Procurement	12
8. Nonconformity of the Technical Specification	12
9. Other	11
10. Administrative Errors and Deficiencies	9
11. Within the Scope of COVID-19 Precautions	8
12. Not comply with the Technical Specifications	7
13. Deficiencies or Errors Regarding the Procurement Announcement	5
14. Procurement Commission Decision for e-Evaluation	4
15. Not Appropriate Administrative Specifications	3
16. Changing of the Procurement Procedure	3
17. No Competition	3
18. Noticing the Missing of Procurement Documents Outside the Announcement, Technical, and Administrative Specifications	2
19. Cancellation by Administration upon Complaint	1
Total	330

the administration may cancel the procurement within the framework of the Public Procurement Legislation (Tab. 4).

In the list of cancellation reasons for open procedure services procurements, the first place is taken by the reason "The Fact That All Offers Are Well above the Allowance/Approximate Cost for Purchase" with 40 cancellations. As it is known, threshold values are determined according to the approximate cost in Article 8 of the PPL, and the approximate cost is taken into consideration while preparing the announcement period of the auctions. At the same time, the procurement commission provides financial compliance by looking at whether the

Tab. 5. Reasons for cancellation of services procurement (Source: Public Procurement Authority, 2020)

Reasons for Cancellation	Procurement Type and Procedure
	Services-Open
1. The Fact That All Offers Are Well above the Allowance/Approximate Cost for Purchase	40
2. No Tenderer with a Tender for the Procurement	34
3. No Tenderer with a Valid Tender for the Procurement	32
4. Nonconformity of the Technical Specification	12
5. Change in the Quality or Amount of the Procurement	11
6. Cancellation with the Decision of the Public Procurement Board on the Complaint	10
7. Within the Scope of COVID-19 Precautions	8
8. Deficiencies or Errors Regarding the Procurement Announcement	6
9. Not Appropriate Administrative Specifications	3
10. Noticing the Missing of Procurement Documents Outside the Announcement, Technical, and Administrative Specifications	3
11. Administrative Errors and Deficiencies	3
12. No Competition	3
13. Other	3
14. Changing of the Procurement Procedure	2
15. For Administrative Reasons	2
16. Procurement Commission Decision for e-Evaluation	1
17. The Failure of the Tenderer to Sign a Contract	1
18. Cancellation by Administration upon Complaint	1
19. Prohibition / Public Prosecution About the Confirmed Tenderer	1
Total	176

unit price offered by the tenders is lower than the approximate cost or not. If the tender submitted by the tenderers is extremely lower than the approximate cost prepared by the administration, according to Article 38 of the PPL No. 4734, the tenderers accept or reject the tender by requesting a written explanation about their tenders. What is generally important here is that tenderers higher than the approximate cost may cause public loss, and tenders lower than the approximate cost may contain unqualified content that does not comply with the technical specification. However, the procurement commission may make contrary decisions because the urgency of the work to be procured may over-shadow the high or extremely low tender amount offered by the tenderers. In such cases, the tender commission decides by taking a risk. However, the pro-curement authority may still approve the decision of the procurement commis-sion under the sixth paragraph of the PPL or to revoke it by clearly stating the reason. Among the reasons for canceled procurements, the second reason is the reason "No Tenderer with a Tender for the Procurement" with 34 cancellations, and the third reason is the reason "No Tenderer with a Valid Tender for the Procurement" with 32 cancellations (Tab. 5).

In the list of cancellation reasons for construction work procurements conducted with open procedure, the first is the reason for "No Tenderer with a Valid Tender for the Procurement" with 10 cancellations. The second reason is that with 8 cancellations, "The Fact That All Offers Are Well above the Allowance/Approximate Cost for Purchase." The third reason is "Administrative Errors and Deficiencies" with 6 cancellations (Tab. 6).

Tab. 6. Reasons for cancellation of construction works procurements (Source: Public Procurement Authority, 2020)

Reasons for Cancellation	*Procurement Type and Procedure*
	Construction-Open
1. No Tenderer with a Valid Tender for the Procurement	10
2. The Fact That All Offers Are Well above the Allowance/ Approximate Cost for Purchase	8
3. Administrative Errors and Deficiencies	6
4. No Tenderer with a Tender for the Procurement	2
5. Noticing the Missing of Procurement Documents Outside the Announcement, Technical, and Administrative Specifications	2
6. Nonconformity of the Technical Specification	2
7. Procurement Commission Decision for e-Evaluation	1
8. Procurement Authority Decision for e-Evaluation	1
9. Not Appropriate Administrative Specifications	1
10. Deficiencies or Errors Regarding the Procurement Announcement	1
11. Changing of the Procurement Procedure	1
12. Administrative Reasons	1
13. Other	1
Total	37

Considering the cancellation reasons for construction works procurements, it is less than the reasons for the procurement of goods and services. The reason for this can be said that among the reasons for cancellation in purchases of goods, goods will be purchased from the SSO.

There is a statistically significant difference in terms of the reasons for the cancellation variable as a result of the Kruskal-Wallis H test conducted according to the variable of procurement type and procedure (p<0.05). In the Bonferroni correction test conducted to reveal the source of the difference between the groups, Since the number of groups in the variable was three, three comparisons were made, and the p-value was found to be 0.05 / 3 = 0.017. The comparisons were made on the value of p <0.017. According to the results of the Mann-Whitney U test conducted to find the source of the difference, the source of the difference was derived from Goods-Open/ Services-Open. It has been observed that the average score of the goods procurements canceled with the open procedure is higher than the service purchases canceled with the open procedure (Tab. 7).

According to the Mann-Whitney U test performed in terms of Partial Tender Type, there was a statistically significant difference in terms of the reasons for the cancellation variable. Reasons for cancellation vary according to partial tender type. When reasons for cancellation were examined, the average of those that can be given was higher than the average of those which cannot be given (p<0.05) (Tab. 8).

Tab. 7. Comparison in terms of cancellation reasons according to procurement type and procedures (Source: Public Procurement Authority, 2020)

Variable	Procurement Type and Procedure	N	Mean Rank	p	Difference Analysis
Reasons for Cancellation	1. Goods-Open	330	301,92	.000*	1–2
	2. Services-Open	176	223,70		.000**
	3. Construction-Open	37	234,84		

*p<0.05 (Statistical Significance)
**p<0.000 (Statistical Significance)

Tab. 8. Comparison according to partial tender type in terms of cancellation reasons

Variable	Partial Tender Type	N	Mean Rank	p
Reasons for Cancellation	Can be given	271	309,16	.000*
	Cannot be given	272	234,98	

*p<0.05 (Statistical Significance)

4. Discussion

During the COVID-19 pandemic, people lost their jobs due to economic contractions in the countries, newly unemployed people emerged, and many
sectors were adversely affected by this situation (Fernandes, 2020; Nicola
et al. 2020). The health sector is the leading sector affected. Since the uninterrupted maintenance of the services is important, it is a critical issue to examine
the procurements that were tendered and canceled in this process. There is a
noticeable decrease when compared to the canceled procurements in 2020 with
the canceled auctions in the period of 2014–2019. Considering the decrease in
the COVID-19 pandemic process, there is a higher decrease than the decrease
experienced due to the economic effects in 2016.

Looking at the first four of the cancellation reasons of the goods procurements,
it is stated that there are no tenders or a valid tender, the purchases of goods
are made through SSO with the decision of the President, and that all tenders
are much higher than the allowance or the approximate cost allocated for
purchase. Looking at the first four reasons for the cancellation of the service
procurements, it is stated that all tenders are much higher than the allowance
or the approximate cost allocated for purchase, there are no tenders or a valid
tender, and the technical specification is not appropriate. Considering the first
three reasons for cancellation of the construction works procurements, there
are reasons for no tenderer with a valid tender for the procurement that all
tenders are much higher than the allowance or the approximate cost allocated
for purchase, and due to administrative errors and deficiencies. In all three
types and procedures, the most common reason is that there is no tender or a
valid tender. Based on this, it can be said that there are many reasons the tender
did not appear. These reasons can be said among them:

– As a result of the deficiency and error detected by the company in the tender
  document prepared by the administration, requesting an addendum by
  applying to the administration and rejecting this request.
– According to the tender document, the tenderers are excluded from the
  evaluation in terms of qualification criteria as a result of not submitting the
  required documents.
– Failure to deliver the tender offer envelope to the administration before the
  time of the bid and the malfunctions in the postal/cargo transactions, the
  inability of the bidders in the tender, etc.

Another important reason for cancellation is tenders higher than the approximate cost. The tender commission is to exclude the offers higher than the

approximate cost, with the concern that they may cause public loss. When the tender document is subjected to any inspection, legal action may be initiated against the tender commission members and the tender authority because the tender commission members and the tender authority cause public loss as a result of the evaluation of the proposals/offers higher than the approximate cost and the tender remaining in these tenders.

Another important reason for cancellation is the President's Decree. With the aforementioned decision, purchasing the goods or services to be procured through SSO has become mandatory. Therefore, it can be said that SSO has a vital position in the supply of goods of public administrations because the institutions authorized by the Turkish Ministry of Health can benefit from the Health Market established within the SSO. University hospitals are excluded. In this regard, institutions authorized under the Turkish Ministry of Health can obtain medical consumables and human medical products from the Health Market without a tender under PPL No. 4734. As seen in the study, tenders for purchases of goods were canceled based on this decision (State Supply Office, 2020). In fact, it can be said that with such a decision, the supply difficulties that healthcare institutions may experience during the COVID-19 pandemic have been eliminated. However, the cost of canceling tenders should not be overlooked because some expenses can and cannot be calculated in every tender process. Some calculable expenses (such as the advertisement fee) are quite expensive. Therefore, it can be said that the cancellation of tenders with unplanned and unqualified personnel causes inefficient use of public resources and a waste of resources.

In the study, there is a statistical significance in terms of cancellation of procurements where partial tender can be given. In this respect, while the tenders are made open or closed for partial tenders, planning should be done in the process of preparing technical specifications. It can be said that dividing service procurements and construction works into parts is not an effective method, and disrupting the integrity of the work may prevent the efficient use of public resources. However there is competition and price advantage.

Compared to the procurements conducted, the rate of canceled procurements is relatively high. The slowdown and cessation of production during the COVID-19 pandemic can be shown among the reasons for the increase in the cancellation rate in goods procurements. Because of the cancellation of some medical services during the COVID-19 pandemic, the administrations resorted to canceling the tenders. It can be said that the administrations are in a difficult situation in terms of service planning. Unforeseen situations have arisen, and even the administrations have resorted to cancellation because it was seen as objectionable to gather tender commissions to prevent the spread of the epidemic.

Among the reasons for cancellation, errors, and deficiencies stemming from the administration stand out. The inappropriateness of the technical and administrative specifications, which are a part of the tender document, the absence of deficiencies or errors in the tender announcement, the notice of deficiencies in the tender documents other than the announcement, technical and administrative specifications, and the cancellation of the tenders because of some administrative reasons (such as public benefit, disappearance of the need) are being. In fact, these cancellation reasons arise as a result of the deficiencies and weaknesses in the management processes.

Planning is one of the main functions of management. The place of human resources among the resources required for production (labor, land, capital, and entrepreneurs) stands out more than other resources. Human resources are in the primary place in the production of healthcare services because of the human is at the center of the service. Human resources play an important role in providing health services to individuals. Health planners and decision-makers must ensure that competent people are in the right place at the right time to meet the needs of the community and deliver health services at an affordable cost. For this reason, rational policies and strategic planning are required.

References

Ağır, H. & Tıraş, H. H. (2018). Evaluation of health expenditures species in Turkey. Kahramanmaraş Sütçü İmam University Journal of Social Sciences, 15(2), 643–670.

Cao, B., Wang, Y., Wen, D. et al. (2020). A Trial of lopinavir–ritonavir in adults hospitalized with severe Covid-19. The New England Journal of Medicine, 382(19), 1787–1799.

Çelik, Y. (2016). Sağlık Ekonomisi (Health Economics). Siyasal Kitapevi (Siyasal Bookstore).

Cicala, S., Stephen P. H., Erin T. M. et al. (2020). Expected health effects of reduced air pollution from COVID-19 social distancing, NBER Working Paper No. 27135. National Bureau of Economic Research.

Fernandes, N. (2020). Economic effects of coronavirus outbreak (COVID-19) on the world economy (March 22). Available at SSRN: https://ssrn.com/abstract=3557504 or http://dx.doi.org/10.2139/ssrn.3557504.

Koçel, T. (2011). İşletme Yöneticiliği (Business Management). Beta Yayıncılık (Beta Publishing). İstanbul.

Liu, Y., Gayle, A. A., Wilder-Smith, A., & Rocklöv, J. (2020). The reproductive number of COVID-19 is higher compared to SARS coronavirus. Journal of Travel Medicine, 27(2). https://doi.org/10.1093/jtm/taaa021

Livingston, E., Desai, A., & Berkwits, M. (2020). Sourcing personal protective equipment during the COVID-19 pandemic. JAMA, 323(19), 1912–1914. doi:10.1001/jama.2020.5317

Lu, H., Stratton, C. W., & Tang, Y. W. (2020). Outbreak of pneumonia of unknown etiology in Wuhan, China: The mystery and the miracle. Journal of Medical Virology, 92, 401–402. https://doi.org/10.1002/jmv.25678

Mejia, A. & Fülöp, T. (1978). Health manpower planning: An overview. Edited: Hall T., Mejia A. Health manpower planning: principles, methods, issues. Geneva: World Health Organization. (9–30).

Nicola, M., Alsafi, Z., Sohrabi, C., Kerwan, A., Al-Jabir, A., Iosifidis, C., Agha, M., & Agha, R. (2020). The socio-economic implications of the coronavirus pandemic (COVID-19): A review. International journal of surgery (London, England), 78, 185–193. https://doi.org/10.1016/j.ijsu.2020.04.018

Polat, Ö. & Coşkun, F. (2020). Determining the relationship between personal protective equipment uses of medical healthcare workers and depression, anxiety and stress levels in the COVID-19 pandemic. Medical Journal of Western Black Sea, 4(2), 51–58. doi: 10.29058/mjwbs.2020.2.3

Public Procurement Authority. (2020). Procurement statistics, http://www.ihale.gov.tr/ihale_istatistikleri-45-1.html. Access date (AD): 17.09.2020.

Public Procurement Law No. 4734, Official Gazette: 22/1/2002 Issue: 24648.

State Supply Office. (2020). Health market. https://www.dmo.gov.tr/Sm/. AD: 23.09.2020.

Tan, W., Zhao, X., Ma, X. et al. (2020). A novel coronavirus genome identified in a cluster of pneumonia cases—Wuhan, China 2019–2020. China CDC Weekly, 2(4), 61–62.

Turkish Ministry of Health. (2020). Duties and powers. https://www.saglik.gov.tr/EN,15621/duties-and-powers.html. AD: 20.09.2020.

TURKSTAT. (2020a). Health expenditures statistics. http://www.tuik.gov.tr/PreTablo.do?alt_id=1084, AD: 10.09.2020.

TURKSTAT. (2020b). Health expenditures statistics, 2018. http://www.tuik.gov.tr/PreHaberBultenleri.do?id=30624, AD: 10.09.2020.

Wahba, M. A. & Bridwell, L. G. (1973). Maslow reconsidered: A review of research on the need hierarchy theory. Academy of Management Proceedings, 1973, 514–520, https://doi.org/10.5465/ambpp.1973.4981593

WHO. (2020). Statement regarding cluster of pneumonia cases in Wuhan, China. https://www.who.int/china/news/detail/09-01-2020-who-statement-regarding-cluster-of-pneumonia-cases-in-wuhan-china. AD: 10.09.2020.

Zheng, Y., Ma, Y., Zhang, J. et al. (2020). COVID-19 and the cardiovascular system. Nature Reviews Cardiology, 17, 259–260. https://doi.org/10.1038/s41569-020-0360-5

Zhou, P., Yang, X., Wang, X. et al. (2020). A pneumonia outbreak associated with a new coronavirus of probable bat origin. Nature 579, 270–273. https://doi.org/10.1038/s41586-020-2012-7

Asst. Prof. Eylem Bayrakçı

Changes in Working Life during the COVID-19 Pandemic Process and Its Effects upon Employees

1. Introduction

It is not possible to deal the COVID-19 pandemic as just a health problem. The epidemic is also an economic threat to all countries in the world and also an unexpected situation which causes radical changes in working life regardless of its field and scope. To understand and make sense of the effects of these changes in working life upon employees and businesses is necessary to adapt to this unusual working life and to deal with these changes caused by the pandemic.

In the report of the International Labour Organization (ILO) dated June 30, 2020 (International Labour Organization, www.ilo.org, 2020), it is stated that the pandemic has effects of workplace closures, more working hour loses than anticipated, and disproportionate employment against women workers. Of course, it is clear that the pandemic has / will have effects on micro-level businesses and employees, as well as these predicted (actual) effects in working life at the macro level. In this process, businesses had to adopt new working and business methods, and accordingly, workplace practices were out of the ordinary. Of course, employees have had to cope with and adapt to these changes outside of their accustomed working lives.

With the pandemic, when we look at the unprecedented measures and changes that businesses around the world have rapidly taken to protect their employees on the one hand and to ensure the continuity of the work done, it is seen that the change in working life that affected the first and most employees was the transition to telework. Telework / telecommuting is a form of work based on the principle that employees do their work using information and communication technologies in a telelocation (Ölçer, 2004: 54). In telework, although it is essential that employees work anywhere outside the workplace, not necessarily from home, due to COVID-19 measures, it is seen that it means working from home in this process. It is known that the physical work environment is very important for many businesses, especially when considering situations such as learning, training, socializing, mentoring, and cooperation. (Reimagining the office and work life after COVID-19, www.wework.com,

2020). However, it is seen that this situation is relatively more important espe-cially for sectors such as banking, education, training, and tourism, and the social and economic costs of telework are higher. Although it seems that tele-work during the pandemic process is preferred among employees for reasons such as productivity and flexible working opportunity, it is also expected to have potential side effects on income inequality among employees (Bonacini et al., 2020a: 3).

With the pandemic, it is seen that the other change seen in the working life in parallel with telework is that the work teams have to become virtual in order to ensure the continuity of the work (Kniffin et al., 2020: 4). Virtual teams are a group of people operating independently of time, space and organiza-tional boundaries, using technology to achieve a jointly shared goal. (Powell et al., 2004: 7). It's seen that bringing together employees at distant distances (Schmidt et al., 2001).

It is seen that another change experienced in working life during the pan-demic process is the virtualization of management and leadership (Kniffin et al., 2020). Remote management and leadership, is the process by which employees are managed using information and communication technologies (Williams, 2002, cited by Ölçer, 2004, 55). Of course, the most difficult part of being a remote manager or leader is that employees cannot be evaluated in the process of doing their work. In this context, focusing on results and evaluating business results and outputs is recommended as an appropriate method. Of course, in this case, when it comes to virtual teamwork, it may not always be possible to determine how much each team member has contributed. At the same time, it is stated that virtual management can reduce the time to receive feedback from employees' managers (Kniffin et al., 2020:5) and learning opportunities, therefore, it can reduce organizational commitment and increase turnover (Vandenberghe et al., 2019 cited by Kniffin et al., 2020).

During the COVID-19 pandemic, it is seen that changes made in working life are related to the transition to telework in order to protect employees on the one hand and to ensure the continuity of the work done on the other. This situation has caused important changes in education and training institutions as it is valid for all enterprises and all sectors. Similarly, as in all over the world, higher education institutions in our country unexpectedly switched to distance education in one day with the COVID-19 pandemic, and this situation has cre-ated a significant pressure on both students and employees. The COVID-19 pandemic has radically changed the status quo of universities, the way they work and their environment (Gomez Recio and Colella, 2020: 6). Recently, con-sidering the decisions made by universities, it is seen that many universities will continue to provide education with the distance education-based hybrid education model or completely with the distance education model, and academicians and administrative staff will carry out their work with a remote and flexible working model. Moreover, it is uncertain how long this process will continue. For this reason, this new working life may inevitably cause a permanent change in universities. University life is not expected to be the same as before, especially due to preventive measures such as international mobility, the decision of repeat travel restrictions, social distance that must be strictly implemented, and the use of masks. Looking at the studies, it is seen that some studies have been carried out on the transition of students to distance education after the COVID-19 pandemic. However, from the point of view of the academicians, who are one of the important actors of the situation, no study has been found on the effects of changes in the pandemic process and coping methods. In this context, the purpose of this study is how these changes experienced in universities, where face-to-face communication is very important, affect academics and what methods they use to adapt to and cope with these changes. For this, 2 of 15 academicians were interviewed face-to-face, 13 of them were interviewed by phone, and they were asked how the changes in their work lives during the COVID-19 process affected them and what methods they used to adapt and cope with these changes and the findings obtained were presented.

2. Methods

The aim of the study is to reveal how the changes in work life during the COVID-19 pandemic affect academics and what strategies to adapt to and cope with these changes. Depending on this main purpose, the questions sought to be answered were determined as "How were the academicians affected by the changes in their working life?" and "how did academicians cope with these changes?"

Qualitative research method was used in the study. The research focuses on academicians' experiences related to changes and methods coping these changes. Qualitative research method was preferred because it is thought that qualitative research would be more useful in obtaining in-depth information about the case studied. In this context, meetings were held with 15 academicians in September 2020. In the analysis of the data, maxqda18 qualitative data analysis program. The analysis technique is the "inductive content analysis" technique. An attempt is made to reach concepts and relationships that can explain the data obtained in content analysis. Content analysis is an "inductive" approach that aims to reveal the concepts underlying the data and the relationships between these concepts through coding (Sığrı, 2018: 280). Traditionally, content analysis is a research method in which data content is subjectively interpreted through a systematic classification process of coding and defining themes (Hsieh and Shannon, 2005; Elo and Kyngäs, 2008). Content analysis can be used as a method for any type of written text, regardless of how research data is collected (Hsieh and Shannon, 2005; Elo and Kyngäs, 2008). Content analysis contributes significantly to a deeper understanding of human perceptions and experiences. Open coding was used in the study and the study was carried out by two researchers (The author of this study and an academician working in the field of organizational behavior with qualitative data processing experience). Thus, codes, sub-categories and themes were created independently by following the steps of Elo and Kyngäs (2008). According to Elo and Kyngäs (2008), at least two people must analyze and encode the data independently and separately. After completing individual data analyzes, two researchers evaluated the codes and themes until a consensus was reached. The obtained data were defined under codes and themes in accordance with research questions and literature, and were interpreted after a consensus was formed.

In the research, the study group was determined using the purposeful sampling method. In the purposeful sampling method, the participants are selected from those who have knowledge about the subject and have experienced the phenomenon under investigation. Inclusion criteria of the participants in the study was determined as; (1) working as an academician, (2) Being affected by the changes in work life during the COVID-19 pandemic and (3) voluntarily wanting to participate in this research. Thematic saturation principle was adopted in determining the size of the study group (Bengston, 2016), it was thought that the data reached saturation when new themes and categories could not be created and similar expressions were used by the participants. In this context, interviews with 15 academics were completed. Information about the working group was presented in Tab. 1:

Accordingly, 9 of the participants are male. 6 of the participants work as Asst. Prof. Dr., 3 of them Instructors, 3 of them Research Assistants, 2 of them Professors and 1 of them Assoc. Prof. Dr. Participants were informed about the study and it was stated that participation in the study would be on a voluntary basis, they could withdraw from the study whenever they wanted, and descriptive information would not be included in the study. For research, primarily it was received approval from the General Directorate of Health Services Ministry of Health of the Republic of Turkey (08.21.2020 date, 2020-08-17T17_21_57 number), later, from the Scientific Research and Publication Ethics Committee of Isparta University of Applied Sciences an ethical compliance decision was taken with the number 30/5, dated 16.09.2020.

Tab. 1. Demographic information of the working group

Participant	Gender	Title
Participant 1	Male	Asst. Prof. Dr.
Participant 2	Male	Research Assistant
Participant 3	Male	Assoc. Prof. Dr.
Participant 4	Female	Asst. Prof. Dr.
Participant 5	Male	Prof Dr.
Participant 6	Female	Asst. Prof. Dr.
Participant 7	Male	Instructor
Participant 8	Female	Instructor
Participant 9	Female	Research Assistant
Participant 10	Male	Prof. Dr.
Participant 11	Female	Research Assistant
Participant 12	Female	Asst. Prof. Dr.
Participant 13	Male	Instructor
Participant 14	Male	Asst. Prof. Dr.
Participant 15	Male	Asst. Prof. Dr.

3. Results

The findings obtained from the research are grouped under two main themes, the effects of changes in business life during the COVID-19 pandemic, and strategies to cope with these changes, depending on the research questions. Effects were categorized as positive and negative effects, and a total of 10 codes were defined, 8 codes under negative effects and 2 codes under positive effects. Strategies to cope with the effects of these changes were categorized as active strategies and passive strategies, and a total of 8 codes, 6 codes under active strategies and 2 codes under passive strategies, were defined (Tab. 2). Thus, 2 main themes, 4 categories and 18 codes were created in the study.

In the light of the questions asked to the participants, they explained the effects of the changes in working life during the COVID-19 pandemic according to their perceptions. It was seen that all participants perceive these changes as "transition to remote and flexible working" and "distance education model" when "changes in business life" are mentioned and express how they were affected by these changes.

12 participants stated that they experienced inefficiency and low motivation with the transition to telework.

Tab. 2. Effects of changes in working life on participants during the COVID-19 pandemic process and strategies to cope with these effects

	Categories	Frame Codings*
Effects of Changes in Working Life During the COVID-19 Pandemic Process	Negative Effects	Inefficiency and Low Motivation (12) Workload Increase (9) Decrease in the Quality of Education (6) Delays in Works (5) Increased Workload at Home (5) Incorrect measurement of learning outcomes (4) Role Conflict (3) Decrease in time for the family (1)
	Positive Effects	Increase in time for the family (6) Productivity (4)
Strategies To Cope With The Effects Of Changes In Working Life During The COVID-19 Pandemic	Active Strategies	Developing Technological Skills (15) Focusing on Academic Studies (8) More Effort for Students (7) Family Support (5) Social Support (3) Getting Away from Home (2)
	Passive Strategies	Hope for the Future (7) Social Isolation (3)

* The number next to each code shows the number of participants who made a statement about that code.

"I can say that all the work is done remotely, just seeing a screen, and the fuss of preparing lecture notes for students has been academically inefficient." (P1)

"Perhaps my work and my publication decreased because I focused on protecting the health of my family and was worried about spending time with them while talking about the negative scenarios that are constantly given in the news." (P4)

"Inefficient, not motivated why? I guess I said let it stay today, I will do it tomorrow, it is not clear what will happen tomorrow, as long as our health is good" (P8)

Workload increase is another negative effect expressed by 9 participants. Some statements about this are as follows:

"Meetings, events or other activities that were postponed or canceled accumulated later, leading to workload." (P10)

"While trying work flexibly or remotely, we couldn't get our jobs done on time, then they all overlapped. In fact, the job we could do comfortably in a week, it accumulated because we could not go, we had to do the same job on the day we went." (P5)

6 participants mentioned the transition to distance education and stated that this situation decreased the quality of education.

"The quality of the education provided with the distance education has decreased because I do not know whether the child is listening to the lesson in front of me, I seem to be telling myself when there is no interaction, most of the students do not attend the lesson. Look, in a class of 70 students, people attending online classes are 8–10. Naturally, you cannot request participation, you cannot give homework or projects, because some students do not have internet access, they are in a difficult situation. Not everyone's conditions are good. Obviously, it was a period when only weekly lectures were completed. Hence, its quality is discussed." (P1)

"The fact that the lessons were done before in the classroom and then converted to distance education decreased the quality of education and became deprived of the efficiency I personally wanted." (P13)

Delay in the work done with the transition to telework is an effect expressed by 5 participants. For example, some participants said the following about this:

"There were interruptions in the work flow because of the transition from working full-time to flexible-time or alternating work. Some things went very slowly." (P10)
"Not being able to meet face to face with the people we work with, especially in the analysis part of the studies, caused the process to prolong." (P11)

"Since we only communicate with our colleagues in virtual environments and on the phone, the time to do things is slightly longer." (P12)

Teleworking with COVID-19 also caused an increase in the workload at home is another negative effect expressed by 5 participants. For example, some expressions are:

"Since I am at home, my children have always wanted something. So I wasn't working remotely for them, it was more like I was on annual leave. As a result, when it came to the evening, I worked more at home rather than work related things and the day was over." (P6)

"Environmentally, other people thinking that I am not going to work anyway has changed my living standards, especially by increasing expectations from me in the household. To be more precise, I had to devote the time I spent to my studies to house-work, because my family members felt that I had no work to do, thinking that I was not going to work." (P9)

The inability to measure the learning outcomes was also said as a negative effect with the transition to distance education. Some statements about this are as follows:

"Is the student listening or not listening to the lesson? Did he learn? Didn't he learn? We don't know. The exam was held, and 24 hours were given for the questions that were given for an hour before. Identical papers arrived, nothing could be done." (P2)

"I think the most important effect of this change was that the result could not be measured. The students was not able to fully learn the lessons, but it was as if they were successful. In this process, a student who could not pass a course of mine for 5 years, and passed the exam of a course I tested, with a 95 average." (P6)

Role conflict is another negative effect expressed by 3 participants.

"In other words, we used to live our working life at work, our family life at home, and our social life in our social environment. However, with the pandemic, our business, family and social life all are within the same four walls. This distracted my motivation and interest in the job. I noticed that my roles were getting mixed up from time to time." (P12)

Finally, the decrease in the time allocated to the family is a negative effect expressed by 1 participant

"Likewise, it can be said that I neglected my wife and family a little during this difficult process." (P14)

In addition to these negative effects that the participants said, it was said that changes in work life had two positive effects, such as increased productivity and time spent with the family.

Increasing the time spent with the family is also an effect expressed by 6 participants.

"Perhaps the most important effect for me was being able to spend more time with my children and family. I saw that my children are very happy because I am at home." (K8)

4 participants, not going to work during the pandemic increased their productivity.

"I think I can say that my workload decreased a little while I was at home because I am a research assistant, so I could spare more time for academic studies." (P2)

"I can say that my work, which would take much longer under normal conditions, took place very quickly, especially in April, May and June. The journal park (dergi park) statistics show that this process was the same for other academics, so it can be interpreted that the COVID19 epidemic was beneficial, at least quantitatively, to academic studies." (P14)

The answers given by the participants to the question of how they coped with these impacts were collected in two categories as active strategies and passive strategies. In the active strategies category, codes of developing technological skills, focusing on academic studies, making more effort for students, family support, social support and leaving home were formed.

During the COVID-19 pandemic process, it seems that the common coping strategy that is spoken by all participants to cope with the changes they experience in working life is the development of technological skills.

"Most importantly, my tendency to technology has increased. I have learned that every job we have done in the workplace can be done remotely." (P12)

"As a result of a small renovation and addition in the room that we currently use as a study and library, we got ready for lessons. With the advantage of being partially accustomed to distance education, we were able to adapt quickly to the lessons." (P14)
"At first, I learned how to upload data regarding the change." (P15)

8 participants stated that they tried to cope with the changes in this process by focusing on academic studies.

"To deal with the difficulties I faced in my own doctoral studentship, I suppose I worked harder than I think. Not being able to meet with the teachers face to face, not being able to get information by calling the teachers whenever I want, pushed me to study much more. Although this issue may seem like a difficulty, it was actually beneficial for my academic development." (P13)

"I can say that I ignored the impositions of the new normal by concentrating on academic studies. Personally, I could not get up from the table due to academic studies while I was able to go out many days." (P14)

Making more effort for the development of students is another strategy expressed by 7 participants.

"In terms of being an academician, efforts were made to overcome the deficiencies by giving students more homework, research or project work, unlike formal education, along with lectures on online platforms." (P10)

Family support is another strategy used to cope with changes in work life and was expressed by 5 participants.

"Obviously, turning this process into an advantage, spending more time with my family than before, spending time for my baby is the positive side of the process despite all the negativities and makes the process easy." (P11)

It was stated by 3 participants that social support was used as another coping method used in the pandemic process in addition to family support.

"I talked to my friends in this process, yes, we did not go to work, but we continued to work and share information with virtual means, we asked each other how to do remote work and distance education, how the lessons were taught, sometimes connection problems, problems with exams, students had problems that we have not encountered before, the work in this process. I asked my friends because the methods of making have changed, and this made me feel very comfortable. We came together from time to time by taking the relevant precautions, paying attention to mask, distance and hygiene. This situation made it easier for me to adjust to the new normal." (P6)

Finally, getting away from home is another method expressed by 2 participants as another active strategy.

"I realized that I was not in a structure suitable for homeoffice working order and I tried to create a working environment outside, but my lack of obligation caused me to not maintain this order. The fact that the libraries were closed and my workplace was in a remote district made it difficult for me to find a working environment. In order to put my work and student life back into order, I try to create an environment away from home environment that makes it easier for me to focus." (P9)

In addition to these strategies that are said to be actively implemented, some expressions of the participants were categorized as passive strategies. Under this category, there are hope for the future expressed by 7 participants and social isolation codes expressed by 3 participants.

"I do not know how long this process will take, but I think it will not continue like this, so how long it can take, although there are certain changes, I think it will be the same and I will return to my students and the laboratory. When you think like that, it feels easy to cope." (P3)

"Thinking positively hoping that the process is temporary and that it will go back to old times helps to cope with changes." (P11)

"Getting away from social life has been a good way of coping for me, the new way of doing business is remote and I don't have to go outside. Since I prefer to spend time at home and work alone, I turned this into an advantage." (P7)

4. Discussion

The aim of the study was to describe the experiences of academicians regarding how they are affected by the changes in working life during the COVID-19 pandemic and how they cope with these changes.

In this section, there is a situation that needs to be expressed before discussing the findings obtained in line with the purpose of the research. This is the perception of "changes in business life" regarding participant academicians. Because, depending on the purpose of the research, the first question addressed to the participants was "How did the changes in your work life after COVID-19 affect you?" From the answers of the participant academicians to this open-ended question, their perceptions about what the changes in business life are can also be defined.

According to this, while the participant academicians talked about their experiences about how they were affected by the changes in working life, it was seen that they mostly focused on the teleworking model and distance education as "change," and they perceived it as a reduction in working hours with the implementation of the flexible working system. In this context, the participants did not mention issues such as the use of masks in their workplaces, social distance, and more attention to hygiene. Indeed, when looking at the studies conducted after COVID-19 in the literature, it is seen that there is a significant increase in working from home (e.g. Akca and Tepe Küçükoğlu, 2020; Bonacini et al., 2020a, Barbieri et al., 2020). Similarly, Bonacini et al. (2020b) stated in their study that in the current context of the COVID-19 pandemic, working from home is the only option to both continue working and minimize the risk of exposure to the virus, therefore it gains great importance for the majority of employees. According to the authors, the uncertainty about the duration of the pandemic and the waves of future contagion even led businesses to see home / remote work as a "new normal" way of working (p.1).

Accordingly, the participant academicians mentioned that the remote / home working model, which they perceive as a change in business life, has more negative effects on them. Inefficiency and low motivation are at the top of these negativities. Some of the participants stated that being in the workplace led them to productivity, but working from home lowered their motivation, so they were inefficient in this new business model they were not used to. Only 1 participant mentioned productivity increase. Another negative effect of remote / flexible working was expressed by 9 participants as an increase in workload, similar to inefficiency statements. Participants stated that they had to do the same job in a shorter time due to the low number of days they went to work in this process, which caused an increase in their workload. In addition, 5 participants also stated that this practice caused delays in the work and business processes slowed down. Working with the findings of Deloitte's (2020) findings gained by using a survey with 334 participants from 17 different provinces in Turkey are overlapping. Although Deloitte's (2020) findings show that the positive effects of home / remote working system on business processes and productivity are proportionally higher, when the data is evaluated on a sectoral basis, the report in question shows that the logistics, construction, education and public sectors' productivity and business processes is negatively affected. According to the comments of the participants in the same study, the negative effects of working remotely include lack of concentration, low motivation due to not being used to such a way of doing business, and it is similar to the findings of this study (www.deloitte.com, 2020: 9). Similarly, Mustajab et al. (2020) stated that working from home was interrupted due to the large number of work to be done at home, thus reducing productivity.

6 of the participant academicians stated that the transition to distance education during the COVID-19 process was a change in working life and said that this situation negatively affected the quality of education. When the statements of these participants are examined, it is seen that there are two reasons for this. The first of these is that students cannot be followed. Academics cannot see the reactions of the students and are not sure whether they are watching the lesson or not. This situation not only disturbs the motivation of the academicians but also affects the quality of their training they provide for. The second reason for this situation stems from the fact that the learning outcomes cannot be measured correctly, and these statements were defined as a separate code as the expressions of 4 participants. Although this finding of the research expresses the views of academics, it resembles with the findings of data by Yılmaz İnce et al. (2020) (same university – Isparta University of Applied Sciences) collected from 1011 students who got distance education in spring term of 2019–2020 academic year in COVID-19 pandemic process. The researchers found that the students were not satisfied with the image and sound quality of the live lessons. Again, Hebepci et al. (2020), in a qualitative study on distance education with 16 secondary school and high school teachers after COVID-19, some teachers stated that distance education was not as effective as face-to-face education (p. 275).

Another negative effect of teleworking / working from home was the increase in the workload at home (5 participants) and the experience of role conflict (3 participants). Similarly, Crosbie and Moore (2004) stated that especially professional women experience more role conflict in the process of working from home because they see housewife and business woman roles as equal. However, only one participant stated that the time allocated to the family decreased. It is seen that the same participant (P14) stated that remote working change caused productivity increase and even focused mostly on academic studies as a coping strategy. In this context, it is seen that the participant's discourses support each other.

In addition to these negative effects of teleworking / working from home on the participants, 8 participants stated that this situation also had some positive effects. The first positive effect is the increased time spent with the family. Akca and Tepe Küçükoğlu (2020: 75) also mentioned this situation as a positive effect in their study on the effects of working from home after COVID-19. There are studies suggesting that working from home contributes positively to the well-being of family members with the effect of "spreading" by decreasing work stress (Li et al., 2014). Another positive effect of working remotely is the productivity expressed by 4 participants. Participants stated that they were able to work more because they were able to adjust working hours by being at home and not to lose time on the road. P14 expressed this as "Academic leadership, studentship, research and other fields have had an inevitable effect, but in general I think these effects occur because the day saves time by restricting transportation, food and similar activities that are not directly oriented to production." Rubin et al. (2020), they mentioned that working from home can compensate for dead time on the road as a positive element.

How the participant academicians coped with these unusual changes in their business lives was another question that the research sought an answer to. Two categories were created from the answers given by the participants, active strategies and passive strategies.

Among the active strategies, the development of technological skills stated by all 15 participants comes first. This strategy seems understandable, given that new and unusual distance work and education are closely related to technological skill. Akça and Tepe Küçükoğlu (2020: 80) stated that technology-based competitive advantage will gain importance in the digital transformation process.

In addition, participating academicians try to focus on academic studies and spend more effort for students, giving them lecture notes, projects, homework, and making them active and productive. This situation provides an opportunity for them to feel more productive and to utilize time. Other active strategies expressed by the participants include family support and social support. Participants try to adapt to this unfamiliar order with the support of their families and friends, and try to cope with ways such as learning about the process and how they do it. Practices similar to these strategies expressed by the participants are among the recommendations of Deloitte (2020: 13–14) to adapt to the system in their work on organizational resilience to the remote working system. Accordingly, in order to accelerate the adaptation and to continue the process successfully, it is recommended that employees work effectively and in a planned manner, use technology effectively and be accessible to meet with their colleagues.

In addition, getting away from home stands out as a strategy expressed by 2 participants. Especially, it is seen that this situation consists of participants who stated that the workload at home is higher with telework, and that the household's expectations about the house have increased, thus they experience inefficiency. In this context, the preference of these participants to stay away from home as a strategy can be considered as a suitable strategy for increasing productivity and focusing on work.

In addition to these strategies, there are future hope and social isolation strategies, which are considered as passive strategies. The hope that everything will be the same is a method used by participating academics to deal with the current situation. Again, social isolation seems to be a method used by the participants both to protect from the disease and to spend the process more efficiently. Similar strategies Kar et al. (2020) were recommended as one of the coping strategies to protect mental health during COVID-19. Researchers; list methods such as positive thinking, hoping, and praying (p. 205).

Following the announcement of the COVID-19 pandemic by the Turkish Ministry of Health on March 10, 2020, the Council of Higher Education announced on March 12, 2020 that formal education was suspended at universities as of March 16, 2020. Within the scope of COVID-19 measures, universities decided to implement the distance education model in the 2019–2020 Academic Spring semester. At the same time, as in all other sectors, universities have changed their way of working and the way they do business and switched to the telework/ home working model. In COVID-19 pandemic, which does not have a proven reliable and effective treatment, social isolation, curfew and quarantine practices are carried out in many parts of the world, especially for risk groups (such as the elderly, those with chronic diseases) (Uysal et al., 2020: 1187). In this situation, which is perhaps the "new normal," which is uncertain for how long it will last, there is a possibility that the said changes in business life may also be permanent. For this reason, it will be appropriate for employees to adapt to their new business life and to adopt methods that will eliminate the negative effects of changes in business life. For this reason, it is especially important that senior management can meet employee expectations. Considering that developing technological skills is the common strategy of all participants, it will be very important for the senior management to follow the developing technology and to assist their employees with activities such as training and seminars. It is also thought that holding meetings to get feedback from employees and increasing communication will also have an impact on productivity and motivation.

References

Akca, M. & Tepe Küçükoğlu, M. (2020). COVID-19 ve iş yaşamına etkileri: Evden çalışma. Journal of International Management Educational and Economics Perspectives, 8(1), 71–81.

Barbieri, T., Basso, G. & Scicchitano, S. (2020). Italian workers at risk during the COVID-19 epidemic, GLO Discussion Paper, No. 513, Global Labor Organization (GLO), Essen.

Bengtsson, M. (2016). How to plan and perform a qualitative study using content analysis. Nursing Plus Open, 2, 8–14. https://doi.org/10.1016/j.npls.2016.01.001

Bonacini, L., Gallo, G., & Scicchitano, S. (2020a). All that glitters is not gold. Effects of working from home on income inequality at the time of COVID-19, GLO Discussion Paper, No. 541, Global Labor Organization (GLO), Essen http://hdl.handle.net/10419/216901, Access date: 19.09.2020.

Bonacini, L., Gallo, G. & Scicchitano, S. (2020b). Working from home and income inequality: Risks of a "new normal" with COVID-19. Journal of Population Economics. https://doi.org/10.1007/s00148-020-00800-7

Crosbie T. & Moore, J. (2004). Work–life balance and working from home. Social Policy & Society, 3(3), 223–233. DOI:10.1017/S1474746404001733

Deloitte, İşin geleceği: Uzaktan çalışma sisteminde organizasyonel dayanıklılığı korumak, https://www2.deloitte.com/content/dam/Deloitte/tr/Documents/human-capital/isin-gelecegi-uzaktan-calisma-sisteminde-organizasyonel-dayanikliligi-korumak.pdf, Nisan 2020, Access date: 20.09.2020.

Elo, S. & Kyngäs, H. (2008) The qualitative content analysis process. Journal of Advanced Nursing, 62(1), 107–115. doi: 10.1111/j.1365-2648.2007.04569.x

Gomez Recio, S. & Colella, C. (2020). The world of higher education after COVID-19 how COVID-19 has affected young universities, Yerun Young European Research Universities, Yerun Brussels Office.

Hebebci, M. T., Bertiz, Y., & Alan, S. (2020). Investigation of views of students and teachers on distance education practices during the coronavirus (COVID-19) pandemic. International Journal of Technology in Education and Science (IJTES), 4(4), 267–282.

Hsieh, H. F. & Shannon, S. E. (2005). Three approaches to qualitative content analysis. Qualitative Health Research, 15(9), 1277–1288. doi: 10.1177/1049732305276687

International Labour Organisation (ILO). (30 June 2020). ILO monitor: COVID-19 and the world of work. Fifth edition Updated estimates and analysis,

https://www.ilo.org/wcmsp5/groups/public/@dgreports/@dcomm/
documents/briefingnote/wcms_749399.pdf, Access date: 20.09.2020.

Kar, S. K., Yasir Arafat, S. M., Kabir, R., Sharma, P., Shailendra, K., & Saxena,
S. K. (2020). Chapter 16 Coping with mental health challenges during
COVID-19, S. K. Saxena (ed.), Coronavirus disease 2019 (COVID-19),
medical virology: From (199–213) pathogenesis to disease control, https://
doi.org/10.1007/978-981-15-4814-7_16

Kniffin, K. M., Narayanan, J., Anseel, F., Antonakis, J., Ashford, S. J., Bakker,
A. B., ... & Creary, S. J. (2020). COVID-19 and the workplace: Implications,
issues, and insights for future research and action. Working Paper 20–127,
Publication of Harvard Business School. doi: 10.31234/osf.io/gkwme

Li, J., Johnson, S., Han, W., Andrews, S., Strazdins, L., Kendall, G., & Dockery,
A. (2014). Parents' non-standard work schedules and child wellbeing: A
critical review of the literatüre. Journal of Primary Prevention, 35(1), 53–73.
doi: 10.1007/s10935-013-0318-z

Mustajab, D., Bauw, A., Rasyid, A., Irawan, A., Akbar, M. A., & Hamid, M.
A. (2020). Working from home phenomenon as an effort to prevent
COVID-19 Attacks and its impacts on work productivity. The International
Journal of Applied Business, 4(1), 13–21. http://dx.doi.org/10.20473/tijab.
V4.I1.2020.13-21

Ölçer, F. (2004). Uzaktan yönetim: Yeni bir yönetim yaklaşımı. Yönetim ve
Ekonomi, 11(2), 53–67.

Powell, A., Piccoli, G., & Ives, B. (2004). Virtual teams: A review of current
literature and directions for future research. The DATA BASE for Advances
in Information System, 35(1), 6–36. doi: 10.1145/968464.968467

Reimagining work in the era of COVID-19, 16 June 2020, https://www.wework.
com/ideas/growth-innovation/reimagining-work-in-the-era-of-covid-19,
Access date: 20.09.2020.

Rubin, O., Nikolaeva, A., Nello-Deakin, S., & te Brömmelstroet, M. (2020). What
can we learn from the COVID-19 pandemic about how people experience
working from home and commuting?. Centre for Urban Studies, University
of Amsterdam. Available at: https://urbanstudies.uva.nl/content/blog-series/
covid-19-pandemic-working-from-home-and-commuting.html.

Schmidt, J. B., Montoya-Weiss, M. M., & Massey, A. P. (2001). New product
development decision-making effectiveness: Comparing individuals, face-
to-face teams, and virtual teams. Decision Sciences, 32(4), 575–600. https://
doi.org/10.1111/j.1540-5915.2001.tb00973.x

Sığrı, Ü. (2018). Nitel araştırma yöntemleri. Beta Basım Yayın Dağıtım A.Ş.

Uysal, B., Demirkıran, M., & Yorulmaz, M. (2020). Assessing of factors effecting COVID-19 mortality rate on a global basis. Turkish Studies, 15(4), 1185–1192. https://dx.doi.org/10.7827/TurkishStudies.44390

Vandenberghe, C., Landry, G., Bentein, K., Anseel, F., Mignonac, K., & Roussel, P. (2019). A dynamic model of the effects of feedback-seeking behavior and organizational commitment on newcomer turnover. Journal of Management. Advance online publication. http://dx.doi.org/10 .1177/0149206319850621

VERBI Software, 2018. MAXQDA 18 (computer software). Berlin, Germany: VERBI Software.

Williams, V. (2002). Virtual leadership. Edison, NJ: Shadowbrook Publishing.

Yılmaz İnce, E., Kabul, A., & Diler, İ. (2020). Distance education in higher education in the COVID-19 pandemic process: A case of Isparta Applied Sciences University. International Journal of Technology in Education and Science (IJTES), 4(4), 343–351.

Res. Asst. Alptuğ Aksoy

The Effect of the COVID-19 Pandemic Process on Organizational Behavior Variables: A Systematic Review Study

1. Introduction

Organizations face uncertainty continually when they meet today's "grand challenges" or serious problems that are generally not restricted to national, financial, or social borders (Carnevale and Hatak, 2020: 183). These difficulties are complex problems that cannot be easily overcome and require innovative ideas such as hunger, famine, war, poverty, and epidemic or pandemic diseases (Eisenhardt, 2016: 1113). Also, they can threaten the survival and sustainability of current institutions and organizations, reorganize their business environment, and affect the management of employees' organizational behavior. Today's grand challenge is the COVID-19 pandemic (Carnevale and Hatak, 2020: 183).

A total of five epidemics have occurred in the world for nearly a century, along with the COVID-19 outbreak. These four pandemics are the "Spanish Flu" in 1918, the "Asian Flu" in 1957, the "Hong Kong Flu" in 1968, and the "Swine Flu" in 2009, respectively (Açıkgöz and Günay, 2020: 520). The fifth pandemic is COVID-19, the novel coronavirus that was announced by the authorities in Wuhan City (Republic of China) in December 2019, later referred to as SARS-CoV-2 (World Health Organization, 2020: 2). This pandemic spread to more than one hundred and fourteen countries before it was declared by WHO as a COVID-19 outbreak on March 11, 2020 (Anjorin, 2020: 199).

As a result of the rapid spread of the disease in the world countries, over 22 million COVID-19 cases and 781 000 deaths have been reported since December 2019 (European Centre for Disease Prevention and Control, 2020: 1). Besides the burden of death and disease, it is a global phenomenon that already has an unprecedented effect on economies and communities (United Nations Development Programme, 2020: 4). The pandemic impacts international economic development unlike anything else experienced nearly a century ago. According to projections, the virus could slash global economic growth by 3.0 % to 6.0 % by 2020. With this economic recession, unemployment rates are expected to increase until the end of the year that has not been felt since the Great

Depression of the 1930s. Also, global trade is expected to decline from 13 % to 32 %. In briefly, the world economy will deteriorate day by day during the pandemic (Jackson et al., 2020: 2).

Global pandemic effects should not be considered limited only on an economic scale. It also has an impact on the social facet of life. To prevent the rapid spread of COVID-19, countries have taken a variety of public health policies, including social distancing and movement restrictions. Schools, businesses, foundations, and associations in the society were temporarily closed due to social distance. Also, public meetings and mass service purchases are prohibited. In general, only the urgent needs of citizens have been tried to be met in many countries. Besides, travel bans were imposed within the scope of mobility restrictions (Brodeur et al., 2020: 2).

In addition to these mobility and travel restrictions, the new lifestyle that emerged with the measures introduced also had significant effects on businesses. For example, most of the institutions in the service sector, such as some wholesale and retail outlets, construction firms, hospitality businesses, and restaurants, have been temporarily closed. Schools in the education sector have started to provide their services online. So this situation reduced the revenues of the organizations and brought them to the brink of bankruptcy (United Nations, 2020: 11).

Of course, these changes in workplaces have also affected the workforce in organizations. Employees have been transformed into either "home-to-work" workers or "life-sustaining" workers (e.g., medical staff), or employees who are furloughed or laid off (Kniffin et al., 2020: 4). Besides, the labor supply is decreasing due to quarantine measures and a decrease in economic activities. Employment impacts have also resulted in a considerable loss of income for employees. This loss of income means less consumption of goods and services that can damage the continuity of businesses and the resilience of economies (International Labour Organization, 2020: 5).

In addition to the impacts of COVID-19 on the overall business and economy, the pandemic is likely to have various social and psychological costs for individuals, including those who have lost their jobs and those who remain employed (Kniffin et al., 2020: 13). Most managers have reduced the number of people working in the workplace. Some of the staff and those with chronic illnesses were sent home for a while. However, business managers still want to ensure the continuity of business during this pandemics, which is thought to be effective in a certain period. Ultimately, employees whose jobs' that cannot be done from home must be at their workplaces. Many new practices, such as measuring the temperature at the door, using masks, and reducing the number of employees working together have been implemented for those staff. In this context, how the COVID-19 pandemic is reflected in the organizational behavior of the personnel working in organizations is an important issue that should be emphasized (Aksoy and Mamatoğlu, 2020: 27).

The COVID-19 pandemic arises as a frustrating and even painful experience, which requires people to understand the current situation and seek suitable measures to cope with the problems (Guan et al., 2020: 1). For instance, the complexity and confusion of COVID-19 have forced companies to intervene to protect the health and well-being of employees. The most common problems faced by employees in this uncertain period are stress, physical and mental health problems, burnout, job dissatisfaction, and organizational performance decline. In addition, it can be observed that individuals become alienated from their organizations due to drug addiction, depression, anxiety. Besides this, the pressures created by the increase in workload, and consequently, cause an increase in employees' intention to quit (Kniffin et al., 2020: 15–18).

Investigating the impact of the COVID-19 pandemic on the organizational behavior variables mentioned above in a single study is essential in terms of the managers to create interventions to reduce possible negative organizational results. Moreover, researching the effects of the pandemic on organizational attitudes and behaviors will provide evidence-based information on the damages of this disease to businesses. However, no such study has been encountered in the literature so far. Therefore, in this study, the effect of the pandemic process on factors, determinants, and predictors that affect the psychological structure and behavioral processes in the workplace was examined.

2. Methods

In this review, the effect of COVID-19 was examined in terms of variables frequently encountered in the organizational behavior literature. Web of Science, Scopus, and Google Scholar databases were used for data collection. As keywords, COVID-19, coronavirus, or SARS-COV-2 were used to investigate the researches on outbreak. The organizational behavior variables with the most frequently used forms in the literature were written together with keywords related to the COVID-19 pandemic and each of them was examined separately.

Only English-language journal articles with full-text are included, and review studies are excluded. However reference sections of reviews have also been checked to ensure that most of the published articles have been reached. Also studies showing non-quantitative results were not included in the study. Initial experiments containing less than 50, due to insufficient sample measurements, were omitted. Finally, a total of 38 quantitative studies have been included in this research.

3. Result

In this part of the study, there is information about the important results of the articles obtained using the methodology. In the study, the relationships between organizational behavior variables such as job satisfaction, organizational commitment, burnout, leadership, intention to leave, stress, communication, anxiety, productivity, presenteeism, job crafting, and COVID-19 were examined.

3.1. COVID-19 and Job Satisfaction

There have been many studies that consistently correlate the occurrence of pandemic outbreaks and a range of psychological and behavioral outcomes (Restubog et al., 2020: 1). Some of these studies are aimed at determining the job satisfaction levels of the employees, which are directly related to the effectiveness and efficiency of the policies created, especially in times of crisis. Job satisfaction examines the awareness and assessment, mental state, and emotional perception of an employee's work and all associated aspects or dimensions (Yu et al., 2020: 2). Employment satisfaction is a vital driving tool for avoiding negative organizational behavior during the outbreak. (Zhang et al., 2020a: 145).

In a study on a total of 304 healthcare workers working in public and private sectors in Iran conducted by Zhang et al. (2020b), it was determined that COVID-19 affects the job satisfaction of employees. However, in this study, it was concluded that the job satisfaction of employees who are not known to have COVID-19 disease is lower than those who are COVID-19 positive and negative.

In the early days of the COVID-19 quarantine, a study conducted on 220 top 15 pharmaceutical companies in Malaysia, where the effect of being an authentic leader on job stress and job satisfaction was examined, revealed that authentic leadership had a positive effect on job satisfaction and a negative effect of job stress (Sultana, 2020: 1836).

Another study conducted on 240 healthcare workers in Bolivia by Zhang et al. (2020c), it was investigated whether the number of office day and age affect the job satisfaction of health staff. At the end of the analysis, it was concluded that the number of days employees worked negatively affected the job satisfaction of young healthcare workers and positively influenced the older healthcare workers.

In a study conducted by Ren et al. (2020), the relationship of employees' job crafting on job satisfaction and creative work behavior was examined among a total of 311 employees from six manufacturing enterprises in China during COVID-19. The findings revealed that job engagement has a mediating role in the positive effect of job crafting on job satisfaction, and age has a moderator role in this relationship.

Labrague and De Los Santos (2020) investigated the effect of COVID-19 fear on job satisfaction, stress, intention to leave the job, and the organization on nurses (n = 261) in five hospitals in the Philippines. They concluded that their job satisfaction levels were high. In this study, they also concluded that the fear of COVID-19 negatively affected the job satisfaction level of nurses.

Generally, employees in an organization prefer a pleasant working environment. For managers, this situation and satisfying the demands and needs of employees can be costly. However, studies show that employees with higher job satisfaction during the pandemic are more resistant to crisis and stock fluctuations. For this reason, in the COVID-19 pandemic, trying to ensure the satisfaction of the employees from the job and the workplace is important in terms of the survival, continuity of the workplace, and increasing its value (Shan and Tang, 2020: 1).

3.2. COVID-19 and Organizational Commitment

Coronavirus (COVID-19) has changed the world's markets and has created more tension and confusion in job relations. In reaction to the epidemic, policymakers have advised people to work from home and to restrict social contact to minimize the spread of the virus. However, while some workers could efficiently work from home due to the nature of their jobs, some employees still had to go to work. This situation has affected the commitment of employees to their jobs and organizations (Machokoto, 2020: 516).

In general, studies show that employees' loyalty to their organizations increases during unexpected disasters such as COVID-19. For example, a worldwide study conducted regularly by Gallup found that 38 % of employees were more committed to their jobs during this period. This finding is the highest value of Gallup, which has made evaluations since 2000. On the other hand, it was determined that 13 % of employees lost their commitment to the organization during the pandemic period (Harter, 2020a: 1)

Regarding to organizational royalty, in three case studies conducted by Machokoto (2020) in the UK, it was determined that COVID-19 affected employees' organizational commitment, especially continuance commitment. In the study, it was stated that employees' loyalty increased due to the need to pay their bills and fear of borrowing. However, it has been found that, in general, during the high-risk pandemic period, employees' love of work decreases.

During the pandemic period, the element affecting the organizational commitment of the employees is the work-related factors. The findings of one study have demonstrated that the corporate climate affects loyalty to organizations. In a study conducted by Athar (2020) on 59 employees in Indonesia, it can be said that the level of piety, resilience, and a great sense of responsibility among the organizational cultural elements of the employee determined his/her commitment to the organization he/she worked in. Other corporate culture factors, such as responsive and competent, have no major impact on the engagement to the job.

In another study conducted in Indonesia, Adhitama and Riyanto (2020) investigated the factors affecting the organizational commitment of employees in the financial sector. In this research, they stated that during the pandemic period, most of the employees realized that they were valued and respected their work and their opinions were necessary for their manager or supervisor. Findings also show that commitment can be affected by social cohesion, feeling supported by the person's manager, sharing information, shared goals, shared vision, communication and trust.

Some facets of the workforce may have a detrimental effect on participation, such as administrative problems, conflicts, management strategy, lack of resources, role conflict and heavy workloads. While it is important to look at these things, we should also concentrate on driving dedication, in particular, growing employee capital and fostering well-being. For example, leadership has a positive influence on commitment, especially through encouragement and feedback (Australian Psychological Society, 2020: 2).

In addition, employees generally determine their commitment to the workplace, organizational policies, leader behavior and various practices. Identifying these reasons for commitment is valuable in terms of organizational results. The performance of the employees and their compliance with the organization are realized much more. In addition, these employees have better problem solving and decision-making techniques. In an environment of competition and uncertainty, commitment plays a major role in gaining an advantage over competitors. As a result, in the time of COVID-19, it is extremely important to manage the level of commitment of employees and determine what factors affect this level (Adhitama and Riyanto, 2020: 8)

3.3. COVID-19 and Burnout

Another organizational behavior variable that is affected by the COVID-19 pandemic is the employee's burnout level. Burnout syndrome was discovered in the early 1970s and is described as excessive use of energy and resources that cause emotional stress or decreased performance (Talaee et al., 2020: 5). While employee burnout levels are significant in every period of business life, this syndrome will inevitably become much more critical in a situation that develops suddenly like COVID-19 and affects businesses almost all over the world. Because burnout syndrome affects the important organizational results like communication, job satisfaction, intention to stay, and organizational commitment and performance of employees. Also, it causes health problems such as headaches, muscle strain, chronic fatigue, hypertension, a sleeping disorder (Zhang et al., 2020b: 1).

In a study conducted by Zhang et al. (2020c), it was concluded that COVID-19 affects the burnout levels of employees (n = 308) in 53 different cities of China. Also, it was determined that the burnout levels of employees decreased as they moved away from Wuhan, but after a certain distance (1020 km), burnout increased again due to COVID-19.

Another study conducted by Barello et al. (2020) on healthcare workers, it was found that the burnout levels of healthcare workers were high in five weeks after the COVID 19 case was seen in Italy. Researchers also indicated that one-third of healthcare workers had emotional exhaustion and one fourth had depersonalization. The study also showed that having symptoms of the disease increased the level of burnout of healthcare workers.

The other study among physicians working at the European Society of Intensive Care Medicine (n = 1001) conducted by Azoulay et al. (2020), it was found that more than half of the physicians have experienced burnout syndrome since the onset of the COVID-19 pandemic. The factors that trigger burnout are age and the perception of the ethical climate in the hospital.

Wu et al. (2020) compared the frequency of burnout among healthcare staff working in frontline and usual services (n=190) during the COVID-19 Outbreak in Wuhan. They found that frontline health workers had fewer burnout levels than usual ward workers. This situation has been explained by the fact that frontline workers have a greater sense of control over their patients' condition, are closer to key decision-makers, and have access to the right information in a short time.

Giusti et al. (2020) also found that 35.7 % of the workers were burnout in Italy (n = 330). In addition, it was determined that the predictors of burnout were working hours, psychological disturbances, fear of infection, and perceived support by friends in that study. Burnout was higher among female employees, nurses, hospital workers, and those in contact with COVID-19 patients.

Most definitely, there was a lack of knowledge and understanding of the disease. Due to the lack of knowledge of the disease, physical and mental problems occurred more frequently among employees during the pandemic. Physical problems are problems such as fatigue, stomach, and intestinal pain, insomnia, muscle cramps. These mental health problems may be generated by a failure to work appropriately, manage and make decisions, and the lack of an optimal ethical climate. As a result, it is normal for employees to experience burnout syndrome due to increased workload and physical and mental problems. In this period, managers are required to make evaluations in terms of the dimensions of burnout in addition to the decisions they make about the disease (Azoulay et al., 2020: 7). Indeed, managers need more knowledge about nature and the underlying causes of this issue to plan adequately for possible outbreaks of infectious diseases and implement appropriate approaches and strategies to avoid this terrible situation further (Jalili et al., 2020: 5).

3.4. COVID-19 and Leadership

COVID-19 can only be seen as a test for countries, leaders, and leadership theory. Everything known in the world has been reversed and these changes will not be restored as soon as possible. What we need in this period is leaders who can defeat the virus and calm us down (Grint, 2020: 5).

However, it is not easy to be a good leader in times of pandemics, and individual and system-related weaknesses in leadership skills can be seen in this period. Moreover, the good things do seem to have positive effects on a variety of lives and it is not clear what these effects will have in the long term. For these reasons, management science had severe problems in performing this most important function at the time of COVID-19 (Wilson, 2020: 290).

In times of crisis such as the COVID-19 pandemic, it is important what management style to adopt. Bartsch et al. (2020) conducted a research on how to lead successfully under challenging periods where service personnel primarily work in simulated environments. Results revealed that managed and enabling leadership behaviors were required in a simulated environment in crisis situations to sustain the role of service staff results. Also, findings showed that the flexibility of the workplace and team cohesion had a mediating role between leadership style and the workplace's performance.

A meta-analysis by Gallup has identified that management strategies will be used to explain priorities, analyze resource and equipment demands and change tasks so that individuals can use their power in different ways. According to the results of a survey of what kind of leader employees need, 39 % of US employees stated that the leader had given them a clear action plan, and 48 % of employees strongly agreed that their supervisor informed them of what was happening in the organization (Harter, 2020b: 1)

The pandemic period has once again demonstrated how significant leadership behavior is. Employees are seeking visible leadership in this turbulent period, in addition to actions taken in their organizations to address concerns over COVID-19. Leaders may need to think of new ways to lead and connect with their teams by paying attention to social distance. Leaders' understanding of employees' sources of concern, awareness of employees' concerns, and development of approaches that alleviate concerns as much as possible will make it easier to overcome this period (Shanafelt et al., 2020: 2134).

3.5. COVID-19 and Intention to Leave

COVID 19 has seriously affected the working styles that employees are accustomed to. Some employees, such as healthcare workers, supermarket workers and restaurant employees, were forced to continue their duties with a higher workload. Some employees were confined to home and started working at home. As both situations are new to employees, they have led to reluctant work, reduced work quality and productivity, and increased intention to leave. Among these organizational consequences, the most costly and painful situation is the intention of the qualified employee to quit (Li et al., 2020: 2).

During pandemic periods, organizations need to measure their employees' intention to work and leave their jobs. For example, in a study conducted by Jang et al. (2020) on 441 hospital workers working in South Korea, it was found that 60 % of the respondents were willing to work in the hospital during an infectious disease epidemic, while 12.5 % did not want to accept the work. In addition, 8 % of respondents reported that they were considering quitting their jobs. 54.4 % perceived their work to be dangerous, and half perceived the severity of COVID-19 as high. The effectiveness of the hospital intervention and the perceived threat level was correlated with the intention of the hospital staff to quit to job.

After determining the level of working and quitting intentions of employees, it is necessary to determine the factors affecting their intention to quit. Hoang et al. investigated why teachers started working outside their home countries due to COVID 19. The research was conducted on 304 teachers working in South Asia. As a result of the findings obtained, it was concluded that the newly arrived country, income and education level were effective in the intention of teachers to quit. Accordingly, living in Thailand and Philippines increase in income and increase in education level are listed among the factors that affect teachers' intention to quit.

A study on factors influencing the intention to leave was also conducted by Yáñez et al. (2020). This study aims to measure the anxiety, stress and turnover intention of 303 healthcare workers working in 11 healthcare institutions in 24 provinces in Peru. According to the findings obtained from the study, it was found that there is a negative relationship between age and the intention to leave the job, and as age increases, people do not want to leave the job. It was also found that healthcare workers in the private sector had a higher intention to quit than those in the public sector. However, gender, education level and employment level and intention to quit are not related.

Another study was carried out by Zhang et al. (2020d) to determine the factors affecting the intention to quit of healthcare professionals (n=240). According to this study, the number of office days and age of healthcare workers affect their intention to leave. In other words, it has been found that as the number of office days increases, employees' intention to leave the job increases, while the intention to quit decreases as the age increases.

The other factor that affects the intention to quit is the fear of contracting COVID-1 disease. In a study conducted by Labrague and De los Santos in the Philippines among nurses (n = 261) on this issue, it was found that the fear of getting sick affects both the intention of leaving the job and the desire to leave the profession. In this study, it was also concluded that the intention to leave the profession was higher than the intention to quit working.

Investigating the factors that affect the intention to quit as well as its effects will help to take the necessary precautions in this regard faster and more appropriate. For example, Li et al. (2020) conducted a study on nurses working in hospitals in China (n = 1,646), and the mediating role of nurses' intention to leave was investigated. Pathway analysis results showed that the aim to quit is to mediate the interaction between disaster preparedness and the desire to respond to a pandemic.

As can be understood from the above studies, since the pandemic, employees are under so immense strain that many have become worried about their careers and some plan to resign. But the protection and retention of health care workers during a pandemic is imperative (Zhang et al., 2020: 1). To order to satisfy the imminent demands for the battle against public safety disasters, it is important for administrators to get a clear view of the desire of workers to leave and the related causes (Li et al., 2020: 2).

3.6. COVID-19 and Stress

Throughout history people have faced multiple mass traumas and tragedies, and while threats to their mental well-being still follow up these incidents (Polizzi et al., 2020: 59). Likewise, employees show more physical and psychological stress symptoms when they are exposed to environmental restrictions caused by the pandemic with high job demands. For this reason, COVID-19 has severely affected the stress level of employees (Mo et al., 2020: 1003).

The outbreak of COVID-19 increase stress and anxieties, due both to fear and confusion as to how the outbreak affects us socially and financially (US Department of Veterans Affairs, 2020: 1). In a study conducted by Mo et al. (2020) on anti-pandemic nurses (n=180) in China, a positive and significant correlation was found between workers' stress levels and anxiety levels. Moreover, it has also emerged that weekly working hours and anxiety are the main determinants of stress (Mo et al., 2020: 1002).

Emergency conditions such as the COVID-19 pandemic may contribute to extreme stress reactions that raise the likelihood of secondary trauma. Hardiness is a defensive factor, which decreases the risk of detrimental effects including this kind of traumatic experiences. In a study conducted by Vagni et al. (2020) on health and emergency workers (n=140 health care, 96 emergency worker) to identify secondary trauma-causing stressors and reveal the protective power of hardiness, it was revealed that healthcare workers experienced a higher level of stress than emergency workers and that the risk of developing secondary trauma was higher in those who took an active role in the treatment of COVID-19.

In the study conducted by Wu et al. on hospital staff (n = 2110) who were in direct contact with patients during the pandemic and university students (n = 2158), it was found that the stress levels of the hospital staff were higher than students (Wu et al., 2020: 2).

In the study, conducted by Lai et al. (2020) found that 71.5 % of healthcare workers experience stress from COVID-19. This study was conducted in 34 hospitals and 1257 physicians and nurses. It was also found that nurses, women, frontline health staff, and those employed in Wuhan, China, recorded more severe stress problems than other health employees.

In another study by Cai et al. (2020) on doctors, nurses and other health-care workers (n=534), it was determined that the COVID-19 outbreak in Hubei triggered increased stress for healthcare workers in Hunan province. In this study, it was found that nurses experienced much more stress and anxiety compared to doctors and other healthcare professionals. Also, doctors were more upset about performing overtime during the epidemic of COVID-19 than other health professionals. Staff over the age of 50 experienced higher stress compared to other age groups.

The other study conducted by Xiao et al. (2020) on 180 medical staff treating patients with COVID-19 infection, it was found that healthcare workers have high-stress levels. In the study, it was also concluded that anxiety level and social support significantly affect the stress level of employees. In addition, it was indicated that the stress level in healthcare workers has a mediating role between perceived social support and sleep quality.

In addition to its elevated level of infectivity and fatality, the 2019 Corona Virus Disease (COVID-19) induced widespread psychosocial effects by triggering mass panic, societal stress and financial damages. The public understanding of COVID-19 referred to as "coronaphobia," has created numerous psychological problems in various layers of society. The most common name for these problems is stress, and the COVID 19 process has been seriously distressful for both home workers and those who are actively at work. Stressors, such as monotony, disappointment, lack of face-to-face contact with collage, lack of enough personal space at work, and financial losses during lockdowns can potentially trigger adverse mental consequences in workers. Therefore, employees should be screened regularly to assess stress using multidisciplinary psychiatric teams (Dubey et al., 2020: 779).

3.7. COVID-19 and Communication

The COVID-19 pandemic has caused unexpected and sudden changes in business and working life worldwide. These changes have forced businesses and employees to vertically change their operational routines overnight and as a natural consequence of this, managers had to decide and do business under an unprecedented lack of clarity (Sanders et al., 2020: 289). In particular, the fact that white-collar employees start working remotely puts more responsibility on managers in terms of making effective and critical decisions that pave the way of a whole range of communication challenges. As a solution to these managerial problems, businesses and managers have resorted to multi-channel and technology-oriented communication tools such as online messages, video conferencing and electronic mails

In a study conducted on the public relations department (n=444) to reveal the changing communication structure in routine and crisis environments, the mediating role of time pressure and uncertainty was examined and statistically significant effects were found. Moreover, increased pressure from news media, citizens, and employees also have a negative impact on the communicative relationships (van der Meer et al., 2017: 426).

The COVID-19 pandemic has critical effects on higher education institutions as well as in many other sectors. Accordingly, in a pre-evaluation study conducted by Sanders et al. (2020) on university administrators in the communication environment it is found that vice-chancellors, president, deans, heads of departments rapidly starts to use more email as well as other electronic communication mediums. The general focus of these messages are methods of working from home, the process of transition from face-to-face education to online education, general hygiene rules and maintaining social distance, and infection cases within the institution.

Risk communication has become another important point, especially in pandemic periods where significant morbidity and frequent deficiencies in therapeutic measures are experienced with high contagiousness and infection rates. Risk communication has been expressed by the world health organization as a matter of conducting a healthy flow of information, advice and ideas in real-time between experts and people in threats to economic, social and health well-being (WHO, 2020). Well-planned risk communication will help employees regain the level of commitment that was easily lost in times of crisis by controlling their level of anxiety and fear (Malecki, 2020: 1).

3.8. COVID-19 and Anxiety

One of the most critical organizational and individual problems caused by the epidemic is an anxiety disorder. Anxiety is among the incompatible responses that may have an impact on organizational performance. This maladaptive response can make an important and positive contribution to organizational dysfunctions. Managers are expected to respond appropriately to correct this behavior, which is seriously dangerous for both organizations and individuals, during pandemic periods such as COVID-19 (Baruch and Lambert, 2007: 85; Huang and Zhao, 2020: 5).

A study conducted by Huang and Zhao (2020) investigated the impact of COVID on anxiety among healthcare professionals, teachers, entrepreneurs, salespeople, workers, and students (n=7,236). The analysis revealed that during the COVID-19 outbreak 1/3 participants exhibited anxiety symptoms, and this condition was no different between males and females. Career transitions are of particular importance in order to consider the human reactions and responses to evolving COVID-19 stressors.

In the study by Yang et al. (2020) investigated risk factors for anxiety in health-care workers in Hubei province, 29.18 % of all participants had symptoms of anxiety. Compared to doctors, nurses were at a higher risk for anxiety. Another important finding is that healthcare workers experienced anxiety during the epidemic, but many did not receive treatment.

Some studies have investigated anxiety along with depression and emotional exhaustion. For example, in the study of Luceno-Moreno et al. (2020), among the healthcare workers (n = 1422), it was determined that 56.6 % had post-traumatic stress disorder symptoms, 58.6 % anxiety disorder, 46 % depressive disorder, and 41.1 % felt emotional burnout. Risk variables for anxiety and depression were identified as gender, long shift working hours, and concern that he/she and his/her family members could be infected. Another study examining the relationship between anxiety and depression, 79 doctors and 86 nurses participated in. Zhu et al. (2020) found out that the prevalence rates of anxiety and depression symptoms among doctors were 11.4 % and 45.6 %, respectively. Also the prevalence of anxiety and depression symptoms in nurses were 27.9 % and 43.0 %, respectively. Another important finding that emerged in the study is that the gender had a significant effect on the depression and anxiety levels of the employees.

Another study on anxiety and depression levels other than healthcare professionals is the study conducted by Rakhmanov et al. (2020) in Nigeria. In this study, the anxiety and depression levels of academic, non-academic staff, and unemployed relatives of them (n = 69) were examined. As a result of the findings obtained from the analyzes, it was found that women had higher anxiety and depression levels than men. Academic staff's anxiety and depression scores were lower than non-academic staff and unemployed relatives. In addition, there was a significant relationship between anxiety and depression scores.

In addition to the factors affecting anxiety, the effects of anxiety on employees are also important. During the COVID-19 pandemic, people with high levels of anxiety have been reported to have serious sleep problems more frequently. For example, a study conducted by Cheng et al. On pediatric health-care personnel (n = 534) of nine hospitals in Jiangsu province revealed that sleep quality was moderately correlated with anxiety levels. The prevalence of anxiety in pediatric healthcare workers during the COVID-19 outbreak was 14 %. Department, job title, and education status were correlated with the anxiety levels of these workers.

3.9. COVID-19 and Other Organizational Behavior Variables

In addition to the organizational behavior variables whose relations with COVID-19 were examined above, other variables that were less studied were also affected during this pandemic period. These are productivity losses (Van Ballegooijen et al. 2020: 1), presenteeism (Eisen, 2020: 1) and job craft (Ren et al., 2020: 1).

Productivity is the core element for an organization and COVID-19 pandemics also affect the productivity level. Van Ballegooijen et al. (2020) performed research on workers (n=4057) in Belgium and the Netherlands. This study showed that this outbreak causes productivity losses. In Belgium, higher losses of production of working people than the Netherlands have been recorded. Participants with babies, youth respondents, and staff with a COVID-19 infection recorded more productivity losses.

In addition, presenteeism, where contaminated workers with COVID-19 are present during symptoms, leads to COVID-19 occupational risk. When infected patients come to work, they both ensure that their colleagues are infected by spreading the disease and cause loss of productivity (Eisen, 2020: 1). Productivity losses due to the COVID-19 constraints were estimated in the presenteeism (30 %) for Belgium and (35 %) for the Netherlands in a research conducted by Van Ballegooijen et al. (2020) after eight weeks of the coronavirus lockdown. Costs of presenteeism were €27.53 Belgium and for €19.11 in the Netherlands.

The sudden outbreak of COVID-19 also had an impact on job crafting behaviors of workers which means that employees adjust their jobs according to their needs and abilities and thus play an active role in changing their jobs. The study realized by Ren et al. (2020) showed that manufacturing workers who consciously improve their skills will demonstrate greater dedication and creativity in their jobs and be happier with their employment and coping with the organizational changes caused by the COVID-19 pandemic in China.

From all these studies, the effects of COVID 19, which has dominated the world for almost nine months, in the field of business and management have been examined and it has been concluded that it affects organizational behavior the most. At this point, managers' supporting the resilience of individuals and organizations, managing shocks, replenishing reduced resources and creating more sustainable career cultures will lead to more positive behaviors (Verma and Gustafsson, 2020: 256; Hite and McDonald, 2020: 435).

4. Discussion

The COVID-19 pandemic is a significant global health issue that still affects public health and safety. While the pandemic is now ongoing, steps to minimize the transmission of the epidemic have created huge obstacles for people's daily jobs as well as their professions more broadly (Restubog et al., 2020: 1). Organizations have had to change their workforce technically, physically and socio-psychologically, and to carry out previously unexperienced managerial processes in a very short period of time and under epidemic pressure.

The International Labor Organization for example predicts a substantial decrease in working hours globally in the second quarter of 2020, in the range of 10.5 % or equal to 305 million full-time jobs, along with a higher year-end unemployment forecast. It is important to identify how working professionals will remain adaptive to this unforeseen pandemic (Restubog et al., 2020: 1). Therefore, all businesses on a global scale had to design more efficient and resilient ways of doing business. All businesses adjust their strategies to respond to old problems, such as real-time decision-making, labor efficiency, market continuity, and security risk. With the change of strategies in the workplace, employee behaviors also change in order to keep up with these strategies. Since it is not known precisely when the pandemic will be controlled or will end, it becomes difficult to determine the effects on the employment market, labor force and working life (Balcı and Çetin, 2020: 50). However, there are studies conducted to determine the effects of COVID 19 on managerial and professional work life. Most of the studies were carried out on healthcare professionals and especially on nurses. The most basic and critical reason for this is that these occupational groups play a vital role in preventing the epidemic and spreading the infection (Mo et al., 2020: 1002; Wu et al., 2020: 2). However, apart from these workgroups, there are also other employees such as logistics personnel and factory workers who work without a break, especially during the lockdown period. In order to better understand the behavioral and psychological aspects of COVID 19, it is important to continue researches on these occupational groups.

When the researches are examined, it has been determined that almost all organizational behavior variables are affected by this pandemic (Verma and Gustafsson, 2020: 253). With all these drawbacks, COVID-19 brings with it a tremendous opportunity for both managers and researchers to support businesses and deliver operationally viable solutions to tackle the largest global challenge in recent history (Carnevale and Hatak, 2020: 183).

References

Açıkgöz, Ö., & Günay, A. (2020). The early impact of the Covid-19 pandemic on the global and Turkish economy. Turkish Journal of Medical Sciences, 50(SI-1), 520–526. https://dx.doi.org/10.3906/sag-2004-6

Adhitama, J., & Riyanto, S. (2020). Maintaining employee engagement and employee performance during covid-19 pandemic at PT Koexim Mandiri finance. Journal of Research in Business and Management, 8(3), 6–10.

Aksoy, Ş., & Mamatoğlu, N. (2020). Covid-19 Salgın döneminde örgütlerde güvenlik ikliminin iş güvenliği uzmanlari perspektifinden değerlendirilmesi. Avrasya Sosyal ve Ekonomi Araştırmaları Dergisi, 7(5), 26–37.

Anjorin, A. A. (2020). The coronavirus disease 2019 (COVID-19) pandemic: A review and an update on cases in Africa. Asian Pacific Journal of Tropical Medicine, 13(5), 199–203. https://dx.doi.org/10.4103/1995-7645.281612

Athar, H. S. (2020). The influence of organizational culture on organizational commitment post pandemic Covid-19. International Journal of Multicultural and Multireligious Understanding, 7(5), 148–157. http://dx.doi.org/10.18415/ijmmu.v7i5.1626

Australian Psychological Society. (2020). Maintaining employee engagement during COVID-19. Publication of APS College of Organisational Psychologists.

Azoulay, E., De Waele, J., Ferrer, R., Staudinger, T., Borkowska, M., Povoa, P., ... & Pellegrini, M. (2020). Symptoms of burnout in intensive care unit specialists facing the COVID-19 outbreak. Annals of Intensive Care, 10(1), 1–8. https://doi.org/10.1186/s13613-020-00722-3

Balcı, Y., & Çetin, G. (2020). Covid-19 pandemi sürecinin türkiye'de istihdama etkileri ve kamu açisindan alinmasi gereken tedbirler. İstanbul Ticaret Üniversitesi Sosyal Bilimler Dergisi, 19(37), 40–58.

Barello, S., Palamenghi, L., & Graffigna, G. (2020). Burnout and somatic symptoms among frontline healthcare professionals at the peak of the Italian COVID-19 pandemic. Psychiatry Research, 113129. https://doi.org/10.1016/j.psychres.2020.113129

Bartsch, S., Weber, E., Büttgen, M., & Huber, A. (2020). Leadership matters in crisis-induced digital transformation: How to lead service employees effectively during the COVID-19 pandemic. Journal of Service Management. https://doi.org/10.1108/JOSM-05-2020-0160

Baruch, Y., & Lambert, R. (2007). Organizational anxiety: Applying psychological concepts into organizational theory. Journal of Managerial Psychology, 22(1), 84–99. https://doi.org/10.1108/02683940710721956

Brodeur, A., Gray, D. M., Islam, A., & Bhuiyan, S. (2020). A literature review of the economics of COVID-19. No. 13411, Publication of PIZA Institute of Labor Economics.

Cai, H., Tu, B., Ma, J., Chen, L., Fu, L., Jiang, Y., & Zhuang, Q. (2020). Psychological impact and coping strategies of frontline medical staff in Hunan Between January and March 2020 during the outbreak of coronavirus disease 2019 (COVID-19) in Hubei, China. Medical science monitor. International medical journal of experimental and clinical research, 26, e924171. https://doi.org/10.12659/MSM.924171

Carnevale, J. B., & Hatak, I. (2020). Employee adjustment and well-being in the era of COVID-19: Implications for human resource management. Journal of Business Research, 116, 183–187. https://doi.org/10.1016/j.jbusres.2020.05.037

Cheng, F. F., Zhan, S. H., Xie, A. W., Cai, S. Z., Hui, L., Kong, X. X., ... & Yan, W. H. (2020). Anxiety in Chinese pediatric medical staff during the outbreak of coronavirus disease 2019: A cross-sectional study. Translational Pediatrics, 9(3), 231. 10.21037/tp.2020.04.02

Dubey, S., Biswas, P., Ghosh, R., Chatterjee, S., Dubey, M. J., Chatterjee, S., ... Lavie, C. J. (2020). Psychosocial impact of COVID-19. Diabetes & Metabolic Syndrome: Clinical Research & Reviews, 14(5), 779–788. https://doi.org/10.1016/j.dsx.2020.05.035

Eisen, D. (2020). Employee presenteeism and occupational acquisition of COVID-19. The Medical Journal of Australia, 213(3), 140–140.e1, doi: 10.5694/mja2.50688.

Eisenhardt, K. M., Graebner, M. E., & Sonenshein, S. (2016). Grand challenges and inductive methods: Rigor without rigor mortis. Academy of Management Journal, 59(4), 1113–1123. https://doi.org/10.5465/amj.2016.4004.

European Centre for Disease Prevention and Control. (2020). COVID-19 situation update worldwide, as of August 19 2020. European Centre for Disease Prevention and Control Publications.

Giusti, E. M., Pedroli, E., D'Aniello, G. E., Stramba Badiale, C., Pietrabissa, G., Manna, C., Stramba Badiale, M., Riva, G., Castelnuovo, G., & Molinari, E. (2020). The psychological impact of the COVID-19 outbreak on health professionals: A cross-sectional study. Frontiers in Psychology, 11, 1684. https://doi.org/10.3389/fpsyg.2020.01684

Grint, K. (2020). Leadership, management and command in the time of the coronavirus. Leadership, 1–6. https://doi.org/10.1177/1742715020922445

Guan, Y., Deng, H., & Zhou, X. (2020). Understanding the impact of the COVID-19 pandemic on career development: Insights from cultural psychology. Journal of Vocational Behavior, 119, 1–5. https://doi.org/10.1016/j.jvb.2020.103438

Harter, J. (2020b). COVID-19: What employees need from leadership right now. Gallup: March 23: https://www.gallup.com/workplace/297497/covid-employees-need-leaders-right.aspx.

Harter, J. (2020a). Employee engagement continues historic rise amid coronavirus. Gallup: May 29: https://www.gallup.com/topic/employee_engagement.aspx.

Hite, L. M., & McDonald, K. S. (2020). Careers after COVID-19: Challenges and changes. Human Resource Development International, 1–11.

Hoang, A. D., Ta, N. T., Nguyen, Y. C., Hoang, C. K., Nguyen, T. T., Pham, H. H., ... & Dinh, V. H. (2020). Dataset of Ex-pat teachers in Southeast Asia's intention to leave due to the COVID-19 pandemic. Data in Brief, 105913, 1–6. https://doi.org/10.1016/j.dib.2020.105913

Huang, Y., & Zhao, N. (2020). Generalized anxiety disorder, depressive symptoms and sleep quality during COVID-19 outbreak in China: A web-based cross-sectional survey. Psychiatry Research, 288, 112954. https://doi.org/10.1016/j.psychres.2020.112954

International Labour Organization. (2020). COVID-19 and the World of Work: Impact and Policy Responses. 1st Edition, ILO Monitor.

Jackson, J. K., Weiss, M. A., Schwarzenberg, A. B., & Nelson, R. M. (2020). Global economic effects of COVID-19. Publication of US Congressional Research Service.

Jalili, M., Niroomand, M., Hadavand, F., Zeinali, K., & Fotouhi, A. (2020). Burnout among healthcare professionals during COVID-19 pandemic: A cross-sectional study. medRxiv. https://dx.doi.org/10.1101/2020.06.12.20129650

Jang, Y., You, M., young Lee, S., & jun Lee, W. (2020). Factors associated with hospital workers' intention to work in south Korea during the early stages of the COVID-19 outbreak. Disaster Medicine and Public Health Preparedness, 1–17. https://dx.doi.org/10.1017/dmp.2020.221

Kniffin, K. M., Narayanan, J., Anseel, F., Antonakis, J., Ashford, S. J., Bakker, A. B., ... & Creary, S. J. (2020). COVID-19 and the workplace: Implications, issues, and insights for future research and action. Working Paper 20–127, Publication of Harvard Business School.

Labrague, L. J., & De los Santos, J. (2020). Fear of COVID-19, psychological distress, work satisfaction and turnover intention among front line nurses. Research Square, June, 1–18. https://10.21203/rs.3.rs-35366/v1

Lai, J., Ma, S., Wang, Y., Cai, Z., Hu, J., Wei, N., ... & Tan, H. (2020). Factors associated with mental health outcomes among health care workers exposed to coronavirus disease 2019. JAMA Network Open, 3(3), e203976–e203976. https://10.1001/jamanetworkopen.2020.3976

Li, J., Li, P., Chen, J., Ruan, L., Zeng, Q., & Gong, Y. (2020). Intention to response, emergency preparedness and intention to leave among nurses during COVID-19. Nursing Open, 1–9. https://10.1002/nop2.576

Luceño-Moreno, L., Talavera-Velasco, B., García-Albuerne, Y., & Martín-García, J. (2020). Symptoms of posttraumatic stress, anxiety, depression, levels of resilience and burnout in Spanish health personnel during the COVID-19 pandemic. International Journal of Environmental Research and Public Health, 17(15), 5514. https://doi.org/10.3390/ijerph17155514

Machokoto, W. (2020). A Commitment under challenging circumstances: Analysing employee commitment during the fight against COVID-19 in the UK. International Journal of Advanced Research, 8(4), 516–522. http://dx.doi.org/10.21474/IJAR01/10803

Malecki, K., Keating, J. A., & Safdar, N. (2020). Crisis communication and public perception of COVID-19 risk in the era of social media. Clinical Infectious Diseases. https://doi.org/10.1093/cid/ciaa758

Mo, Y., Deng, L., Zhang, L., Lang, Q., Liao, C., Wang, N., ... & Huang, H. (2020). Work stress among Chinese nurses to support Wuhan in fighting against COVID-19 epidemic. Journal of Nursing Management, 1002–1009. http://dx.doi.org/10.1111/jonm.13014

Polizzi, C., Lynn, S. J., & Perry, A. (2020). Stress and coping in the time of covid-19: Pathways to resilience and recovery. Clinical Neuropsychiatry, 17(2), 59–62. https://doi.org/10.36131/ CN20200204

Rakhmanov, O., Demir, A., & Dane, S. (2020). A brief communication: Anxiety and depression levels in the staff of a Nigerian Private University during COVID 19 pandemic outbreak. Journal of Research in Medical and Dental Science, 8, 118–122.

Ren, T., Cao, L., & Chin, T. (2020). Crafting jobs for occupational satisfaction and innovation among manufacturing workers facing the COVID-19 crisis. International Journal of Environmental Research and Public Health, 17(11), 3953, 1–12, https://doi.org/10.3390/ijerph17113953

Restubog, S. L. D., Ocampo, A. C. G., & Wang, L. (2020). Taking control amidst the chaos: Emotion regulation during the COVID-19 pandemic. Journal of Vocational Behavior, https://doi.org/10.1016/j.jvb.2020.103440

Sanders, K., Nguyen, P. T., Bouckenooghe, D., Rafferty, A., & Schwarz, G. (2020). Unraveling the what and how of organizational communication to employees during COVID-19 pandemic: Adopting an attributional lens. The Journal of Applied Behavioral Science, 56(3), 289–293. https://doi. org/10.1177/0021886320937026

Shan, C., & Tang, D. Y. (2020). The value of employee satisfaction in disastrous times: Evidence from Covid-19. Report of SSRN, 3560919.

Shanafelt, T., Ripp, J., & Trockel, M. (2020). Understanding and addressing sources of anxiety among health care professionals during the COVID-19 pandemic. Jama, 323(21), 2133. http://dx.doi.org/2134. 10.1001/ jama.2020.5893

Sultana, U. S., Tarofder, A. K., Darun, M. R., Haque, A., & Sharief, S. R. (2020). Authentic leadership effect on pharmacists job stress and satisfaction during COVID-19 pandemic: Malaysian perspective. Talent Development & Excellence, 12(3), 1824–1841.

Talaee, N., Varahram, M., Jamaati, H., Salimi, A., Attarchi, M., Kazempour dizaji, M., Sadr, M., Hassani, S., Farzanegan, B., Monjazebi, F.,& Seyedmehdi, S. M. (2020). Stress and burnout in health care workers during COVID-19 pandemic: Validation of a questionnaire. Zeitschrift Fur Gesundheitswissenschaften, 1–6. Advance online publication. https://doi. org/10.1007/s10389-020-01313-z

United Nations. (2020). Measuring the impact of COVID-19 with a view to reactivation. Publication of Economic Commission for Latin America and the Caribbean.

United Nations Development Programme. (2020). COVID-19 and human development: Assessing the crisis, envisioning the recovery. Publication of United Nations Development Programme.

US Department of Veterans Affairs. (2020). Managing stress associated with the COVID-19 virus outbreak. Publication of National Center for PTSD.

Van Ballegooijen, H., Goossens, L., Bruin, R. H., Michels, R., & Krol, M. (2020). Concerns, quality of life, access to care and productivity of the general population during the first 8 weeks of the coronavirus lockdown in Belgium and the Netherlands. medRxiv. https://doi.org/10.1101/2020.07.24.20161554

van der Meer, T. G., Verhoeven, P., Beentjes, H. W., & Vliegenthart, R. (2017). Communication in times of crisis: The stakeholder relationship under pressure. Public Relations Review, 43(2), 426–440. https://doi.org/10.1016/j. pubrev.2017.02.005

Vagni, M., Maiorano, T., Giostra, V., & Pajardi, D. (2020). Hardiness, stress and secondary trauma in Italian healthcare and emergency workers during the COVID-19 pandemic. Sustainability, 12(14), 5592. https://doi.org/10.3390/ su12145592

Verma, S., & Gustafsson, A. (2020). Investigating the emerging COVID-19 research trends in the field of business and management: A bibliometric analysis approach. Journal of Business Research, 118(2020), 253–261. https:// doi.org/10.1016/j.jbusres.2020.06.057

Wilson, S. (2020). Pandemic leadership: Lessons from New Zealand's approach to COVID-19. Leadership, 16(3), 279–293. https://doi.org/10.1177/ 1742715020929151

World Health Organization. (2020). Coronavirus disease 2019 (COVID-19): Situation report, 94. World Health Organization Publications. World Health Organization. General information on risk communication. https:// www.who.int/risk-communication/background/en/.

Wu, W., Zhang, Y., Wang, P., Zhang, L., Wang, G., Lei, G., … & Huang, F. (2020). Psychological stress of medical staffs during outbreak of COVID-19 and adjustment strategy. Journal of Medical Virology. https://doi.org/10.1002/ jmv.25914

Wu, Y., Wang, J., Luo, C., Hu, S., Lin, X., Anderson, A. E., … & Qian, Y. (2020). A comparison of burnout frequency among oncology physicians and nurses working on the front lines and usual wards during the COVID-19 epidemic in Wuhan, China. Journal of Pain and Symptom Management, 60(1), e60– e65. https://doi.org/10.1016/j.jpainsymman.2020.04.008

Xiao, H., Zhang, Y., Kong, D., Li, S., & Yang, N. (2020). The effects of social support on sleep quality of medical staff treating patients with coronavirus disease 2019 (COVID-19) in January and February 2020 in China. Medical Science Monitor: International Medical Journal of Experimental and Clinical Research, 26, e923549. https://doi.org/10.12659/MSM.923549

Yang, X., Zhang, Y., Li, S., & Chen, X. (2020). Risk factors for anxiety of otolaryngology healthcare workers in Hubei province fighting coronavirus disease 2019 (COVID-19). Social Psychiatry and Psychiatric Epidemiology, 1–7. https://doi.org/10.1007/s00127-020-01928-3

Yáñez, J. A., Afshar Jahanshahi, A., Alvarez-Risco, A., Li, J., & Zhang, S. X. (2020). Anxiety, distress, and turnover intention of healthcare workers in peru by their distance to the epicenter during the COVID-19 crisis. The American Journal of Tropical Medicine and Hygiene, tpmd200800. https:// doi.org/10.4269/ajtmh.20-0800

Yu, X., Zhao, Y., LI, Y., Hu, C., Xu, H., Zhao, X., & Huang, J. (2020). Factors associated with job satisfaction of frontline medical staff fighting against COVID-19 in China: A cross-sectional study. Frontiers in Public Health, 8, 426.

Zhang, S. X., Chen, J., Jahanshahi, A. A., Alvarez-Risco, A., Dai, H., Li, J., & Patty-Tito, R. (2020d). Succumbing to the COVID-19 pandemic: healthcare workers not satisfied and intend to leave their jobs. medRxiv, 1–13. https://doi.org/10.1101/2020.05.22.20110809

Zhang, S. X., Huang, H., & Wei, F. (2020c). Geographical distance to the epicenter of Covid-19 predicts the burnout of the working population: Ripple effect or typhoon eye effect?. Psychiatry Research, 288. https://doi.org/10.1016/j.psychres.2020.112998

Zhang, S. X., Liu, J., Jahanshahi, A. A., Nawaser, K., Li, J., & Alimoradi, H. (2020b). When the storm is the strongest: The health conditions and job satisfaction of healthcare staff and their associated predictors during the epidemic peak of COVID-19. medRxiv. https://doi.org/10.1101/2020.04.27.20082149

Zhang, S. X., Liu, J., Jahanshahi, A. A., Nawaser, K., Yousefi, A., Li, J., & Sun, S. (2020a). At the height of the storm: Healthcare staff's health conditions and job satisfaction and their associated predictors during the epidemic peak of COVID-19. Brain, Behavior, and Immunity, 87, 144–146. https://doi.org/10.1016/j.bbi.2020.05.010

Zhu, J., Sun, L., Zhang, L., Wang, H., Fan, A., Yang, B., ... & Xiao, S. (2020). Prevalence and influencing factors of anxiety and depression symptoms in the first-line medical staff fighting against COVID-19 in Gansu. Frontiers in Psychiatry, 11. 10.3389/fpsyt.2020.00386

Asst. Prof. Umut Can Öztürk

COVID-19 and Human Resources Management: Primary Reactions, Perceptions and Interventions of HRM Professionals

1. Introduction and Literature Review

Following the report of pneumonia cases of unknown etiology on December 31, 2019 in Wuhan, Hubei Province, China. On January 7, 2020, the World Health Organization identified a new type of coronavirus that had not been detected in humans before. When the first cases detected in Turkey originated in Europe 11 March 2020 48 cases and deaths in some European countries began to appear and the World Health Organization has declared a pandemic on the same date (Özlü and Öztaş, 2020).

With the increase of the case in our country, a series of measures against the epidemic started to be put into effect by the Ministry of Internal Affairs; First of all, primary, high school and university education was suspended, and the activities of kindergartens and childcare centers were stopped. Afterwards, it temporarily stopped the activities of the workplaces in the closed area for social, entertainment and shopping, which will be together collectively. Within the framework of this circular, the activities of 49 thousand 382 workplaces were suspended (Yükseler, 2020). Following these practices, restrictions on public events, extensive travel and transportation restrictions. The temporary closure of places where people are located, football, basketball, handball, volleyball leagues are postponed, Only package service limitations to restaurants, the capacity of public transportation vehicles are reduced to 50 %, the sale of non-essential materials in the market places is prohibited, intercity bus-plane travel is subject to permission and stopping flights abroad (TÜBA, 2020). In the news published by NTV at the end of March, the activities of barbershops, hairdressers and beauty centers were temporarily suspended in the third wave of measures. According to the statements of the Minister of Internal Affairs, the number of businesses closed within the scope of these two circulars reached 211,670 (Yükseler, 2020). In this process, many sectors were affected too much and they had to make unexpected changes in their systems. As COVID-19 affects public health, metaphorically, it has invested the economy in intensive care, which must be treated and monitored carefully in a context. During the process, the HRM system conceived of unexpected transformations and decisions.

In order to survive, today's organizations have adapted to the idea of staying prepared and adaptable with a proactive perspective against unforeseen events and crises that create uncertainty and threaten the performance and sustainability of the organization with the ever-changing environmental conditions. However, with the recent COVID-19 outbreak, all organizations are suddenly compelled to come up with new solutions to the unprecedented challenges that arise in many areas affecting all their functional organs. Many studies conducted around the world show that HR departments play a central and active role in supporting practices to improve business performance as they are directly linked to human resources in times of crisis (Lositska and Bieliaieva, 2020). As Demirkıran et al. (2016) stated in their studies, in the world where today's competition conditions exist, the past perception of the worker has completely changed and lost its importance. The primary resource providing competitive advantage to organizations is human resources. The importance of HR as the unit that processes and manages this resource is increasing day by day. In this context, the perspectives of HRM professionals on the subject, their primary intervention, their perception of the subject has become a topic of interest for researchers. In this study, the premise perceptions and interventions of HRM professionals operating in Turkey on the subject early in the COVID-19 process has been reviewed by detected.

Many new sources of change and pioneers exist with the perception of the individual, accordingly, we know that it is accepted or rejected by saying "New World Order," "New Normal," "New Human," "Post-modernism," "Post-truth." However, a process continues in which every individual in the world is evaluated within the scope of "A New Meaning" by changing its shape with its accessibility (Şen and Batı, 2020). Evaluating the effects that occur in the crisis environment only in a mechanical dimension can cause fatal errors apart from being impossible for today's organizations. The uncertainty, chaos created by the crisis environment and the unexpected situation that creates high anxiety is on the employees; fear, anxiety, insecurity, tension, exhaustion, loneliness create self-defense and overreaction. Crisis primarily threatens the trust of people's basic instincts. When people are threatened with being unemployed and broke, they think their lives are threatened. This situation causes a decrease in the motivation of the employees, and a state of anger, accusations towards each other and communication disorder begins (Akıncı, 2011). At this point, the undeniable importance of human resources management emerges. Because the most important element of an organization is human resources; Unlike other production factors and internal resources, it is the only factor that makes and implements decisions. Therefore, it constitutes the focal point of the success of the organization (Şimşek and Aydoğan, 2000).

In just a few months with the COVID-19 Stage, the world as we know it has changed dramatically as we struggle to adapt to new realities. Work and employee structure changed as employees learned to cope with fast shifts, health problems, financial troubles and domestic difficulties that could be stressful and confusing (Ata, 2020). As Kane (1998) stated widespread thought about, "Human Resources Management policies have assumed an auxiliary role in the realization of organizational change programs and in the implementation of various crisis period policies." has become "human resources management is indispensable and one of the most important functions for any organization in these unprecedented times (Ata, 2020)" with this process. Because with the COVID-19 Pandemic, while organizations continue to make tough decisions to survive and minimize job losses, HR teams organize employees and maintain morale, restructure workflows, reorganize skills and develop staff to help them stay relevant. There have been HR teams tasked with providing the much-needed emotional support to employees while ensuring the continuous productivity of each individual (Ata, 2020).

In Seattle, the center of COVID-19 cases in the USA, Amazon, LinkedIn, Microsoft and Google started working from home in late February. At the beginning of March, Twitter promised all employees around the world to work from home, including hourly employees, with a refund covering the cost of purchasing products such as computer equipment, desks and ergonomic chairs, so that employees can set up home offices. Even in China, where the home-working model is much less common than in the West, local governments and companies across the country have encouraged their employees to stay at home since February 3 (Atasoy, 2020: 1). As the seriousness of the situation increased, not only the market-leading giant companies but other companies had to initiate compliance processes. Because the results of the measures taken and the reflections of the crisis have emerged very quickly. In Turkey, in line with the world, is located along with the announcement of the first case on March 11, many companies and public institutions have made the transition to work from home as a compulsory medium. Although the private sector takes action more quickly than the public sector, they have adopted the full-time home-working model. Public institutions have also switched to a rotational working model in the Presidential Circular published in the Official Gazette on 22/03/2020, provided that they have a minimum number of personnel to meet the needs (Atasoy, 2020: 1).

It is possible to call the COVID-19 Pandemic crisis "unknown unknown" for human resources management. This statement has been coined to refer to a rare and unknown event formalized in economic theory by the American economist Frank Knight (1885–1972); There are things we know which we do not know, we call them known unknowns, and there are unknown unknowns, and these are things we do not know-we do not know yet (Grech, 2020). In other words, the crisis experienced with COVID-19 is a crisis that has not been tested before for the modern world, and its effects have unexpectedly fallen on the human resources management. Misuse of human resources in the event, crisis management and resolution that causes more damage than the actual crisis itself and ignoring many of human characteristics (Weiseath et al., 2002: 36). In this context, In this context, HRM managers have been given too much responsibility. They had to develop sudden reactions to a sudden event. The emergency measures reflected in the literature are compiled and shared from the studies of Atasoy (2020) and HBS (2020) in Tab. 1 under the headings.

As seen in the table above, as Lewis (2020) stated "Not only are HR professionals concerned about employees' health and well-being during the pandemic, they are also under the strain of processing the paperwork and providing solace to the millions of workers who have been laid off or furloughed. For employees still on the job, HR managers are trying to keep their workers productive, motivated, engaged and connected—all factors that are moving targets in the new normal."

At the end of this process, COVID-19 will have permanent effects on HRM. Emergency action plans implemented now will transform into renewed business models. Ata (2020) expressed this situation as "Undoubtedly, the end of the pandemic will bring back a different workforce. The COVID-19 crisis will certainly serve as a case study and blueprint for HR professionals around the world to build effective crisis policies and frameworks. Actions taken now will leave a lasting impact on organizations in a post-COVID-19 world. In sync with management leaders, HR can ensure that the organizations remain ahead of the curve." in his study. When the literature is reviewed, the lessons learned and predicted transformations for the post-COVID-19 process by HR experts, professionals and researchers are summarized as follows (Bingham, 2020; Crawford, 2020; Moncrief ve O'Keefe, 2020; Vazquez ve Puron, 2020; Weggemans ve Bennink-Bai, 2020a; Weggemans ve Bennink-Bai, 2020b);

Tab. 1. Emergency concept changes in workplace practices

Concept	Explanation
Work from Home (WFH)	Working at home (working for wages at home), which has gained importance today with the development of new technologies, is the oldest and most common form of flexible employment that was applied before the industrial revolution (Kayhan Kuzgun, 2007: 4–11). The development of connection and communication technologies has accelerated the tendency to work remotely. Since "remote working" can include working from anywhere, it is more efficient for those who can work individually, such as professionals who need to perform complex tasks that require less interaction (Allen et al., 2014). In this process, work from home / remote work activities have been implemented worldwide in the process that includes health considerations.
Digital Workforce	It is seen that the companies that made the fastest transition to remote work were companies that invested in tools that support virtual work and communication in previous years with the COVID-19 epidemic. At the end of the epidemic, it is thought that not only companies that are currently investing in the digital workforce, but almost all companies will begin to accelerate their investments in communication tools and technology in their long-term and strategic plans. In this process, it is predicted that the behavior of going somewhere will evolve to work remotely (Atasoy, 2020: 1).
Virtual Teams	Structural scaffolds need to be created to reduce conflicts, discipline teams, and ensure safe and complete information processing. Within this, it is necessary to formalize team processes, clarify team goals, and create structural solutions to encourage psychologically safe and efficient exchange of ideas (Gibson and Gibbs, 2006; Huang et al., 2002). In order to reduce the socio-psychological effects of virtualization, it is important to create a team of people with the right number and quality to enable remote work.
Virtual Leadership and Management	It is emphasized that companies that keep their employees' morale high in extraordinary situations, provide psychological support to them and take various actions and measures in this context will increase their values more at the end of this process (Atasoy, 2020: 1). In a collective society and feminine culture features exhibits such as Turkey, in the home / online working order, as the interaction between organization and employee decreases, disconnections occur. At this point, virtual leadership and management skills come into play. While instilling belonging to organization members, keeping them together is challenging even when physically together, it requires more skill and skill in online processes.
Job Security and Continuity	In crisis situations such as the COVID-19 process, companies are recommended to maintain business continuity, stay in contact with customers, understand and support their employees, develop solutions to supply chain problems, strengthen digital competencies and stay in touch with other businesses in the same ecosystem in order to ensure their financial continuity (Atasoy, 2020: 1). When the organization shakes the belief and confidence of the employee in job security, the employee enters the phase of breaking away from the organization and its empathic bond with it. In times of crisis, this is completely a risk factor.

- Fostering positive mental health in the workplace
- Communication Is Critical
- Remote people management: work smarter, not harder
- Keep Your Employees Motivated
- Fast-Tracking Digital Acceptance
- Make employee safety the top priority
- Rethinking Succession Planning
- Focus is largely still near term
- Rewriting the Rules of Engagement Through Camaraderie and Collaboration

The items summarized above are composed of the titles mentioned by the aforementioned researchers and they are indirectly similar. In general, it is clearly seen that HR has been reshaped with COVID-19. It is understood that motivation and basic working principles are shining again, new business models have emerged with digitalization, and these models have brought new unknowns with them, and HR will not be the same again with the new normal. However, the only unchanging point It has been understood that the human resource is a fundamental value for the organization and cannot be abandoned in the short term.

2. Methods

The main objective of this research to identify preliminary perceptions of the issue at the beginning of the COVID-19 process, the first interventions and the changes they feel who are the HRM professionals in Turkey and also to interpret them in a behavioral dimension. In order to determine the perceptions of HR professionals about the COVID-19 process, the relevant literature was first reviewed. Open-ended interview questions were prepared as a result of the literature review. The open-ended questions prepared were presented to the opinion of two academicians who are experts in the field, and expert opinion was obtained. After the expert opinion was obtained, two HR professionals were piloted and the semi-structured interview form was finalized in accordance with the purpose of the research.

The participant group that will serve the purpose of the research was determined in order to collect data with the interview form prepared. Purposeful sampling method was used while determining the participants. In this direction, it was tried to reach professionals working in different organizations, at least at the expert level, in administrative positions in the field of HRM. When the frequency of repetitions was noticed in the information obtained from the participants on the subject, the interviews were ended considering that the "satisfaction point" was reached. The saturation point indicates a situation in which sufficient evidence has emerged regarding the research problem. Researchers who reach this point are recommended to stop collecting data (Yıldırım and Şimşek, 2013). The determined participant group was informed about the purpose of the research and that the information they will give will be used for scientific purposes. In this context, attention has been paid to the voluntary participation of the participants. The participants were told that the interview would take approximately 15–20 minutes and they could finish the interview at the place they wanted.

Since the data collection tool of the research consists of open-ended questions, content analysis was performed in the evaluation of the data obtained and open coding method was used. The data obtained were transferred to the computer environment and the texts formed during the transcription process were carefully read several times and encoded. The codes were explained and interpreted and the results were tried to be presented in line with the purpose of the research. In some cases, the researcher quoted interviews to support the comments and findings. The researcher and a faculty member experienced in qualitative research made separate codes on the data obtained in the interview, and the consistency ratio was calculated by comparing the codes. In this study, the formula for percentage of agreement was used to determine the reliability in content analysis. Agreement percentage was calculated using the formula "Reliability = Agreement / (Agreement + Disagreement) x 100" (Miles and Huberman, 1994). In the study, using this formula, the percentage of agreement in coding; The general agreement level was calculated as 0.85 for the first question, 0.96 for the second question, 0.83 for the third question, 0.87 for the fourth question and 0.88 for all questions in total. Yıldırım and Şimşek (2013) stated in their study that being over 70 % is sufficient for the coding reliability of the researchers.

3. Results

In this part of the study, the preliminary perceptions of HR professionals regarding the COVID-19 process are included within the framework of the data obtained from the interviews.

Considering the age distribution of the participants, it is seen that there is a distribution between 25 and 50 years old. It is thought that the diversity of the distribution will provide an advantage to the research in order to see the holistic perspectives of the x, y and z generations and to see the ideas from

Tab. 2. Distribution of participants' age and years of experience

	Age	Frequency	Percent		Year	Frequency	Percent
AGE DISTRIBUTIONS OF PARTICIPANTS	25,00	4	11,1	DISTRIBUTION OF PARTICIPANTS BY YEARS OF EXPERIENCE IN HR	2,00	4	11,1
	27,00	4	11,1		3,00	4	11,1
	28,00	4	11,1		4,00	4	11,1
	29,00	1	2,8		5,00	1	2,8
	30,00	3	8,3		6,00	2	5,6
	31,00	2	5,6		7,00	2	5,6
	32,00	4	11,1		8,00	5	13,9
	33,00	1	2,8		9,00	2	5,6
	34,00	2	5,6		10,00	2	5,6
	36,00	1	2,8		11,00	1	2,8
	37,00	2	5,6		12,00	1	2,8
	39,00	2	5,6		14,00	2	5,6
	41,00	1	2,8		15,00	1	2,8
	42,00	1	2,8		16,00	1	2,8
	43,00	1	2,8		20,00	1	2,8
	47,00	1	2,8		24,00	1	2,8
	48,00	1	2,8		25,00	2	5,6
	50,00	1	2,8		Total	36	100,0
	Total	36	100,0				

different perspectives. While 17 of the 36 participants are in their 20s, 6 of them are 40 years or older. Depending on this, the remaining 13 of them are in their 30s. Almost in direct proportion to age, their experience in the field of HR also varies between 2 years and 25 years. The effect of age and experience on opinions is another advantage of the study.

When the distribution of the participants in terms of the sectors they work in is examined in the table above, the majority of the "Tourism" sector is seen with a frequency of 33.3 %, followed by the production-weighted "Industry" sector with a frequency of 16.7 %. In the context of the literature, the two sectors, which are stated to be affected the most, take part in the study with the same frequency, will help to look at the current problem from the right angle. Participants from 10 sectors other than the aforementioned two sectors will add value to the work in order to present different perspectives.

When the administrative position distribution of the participants is examined, it is possible to mention the presence of managers in both operational and strategic decision-making positions. 13 experts, 5 Chefs/Supervisor, 3

Tab. 3. Sectors, administrative positions and gender distribution of the participant

		Sector	N	%		Position	N	Percent
ACTIVITY FIELDS OF THE COMPANIES WHICH PARTICIPANT'S WORK		Transportation	1	2,8	**ADMINISTRATIVE POSITION**	Expert	13	36,1
		Tourism	12	33,3		Supervisor	5	13,9
		Automotive	1	2,8		Assistant Manager	3	8,3
		Industry	6	16,7		Manager	15	41,7
		Food Production	3	8,3		Total	36	100,0
		Finance	2	5,6				
		Health	3	8,3				
		IT	1	2,8				
		Logistics	2	5,6		**Gender**	**N**	**Percent**
		Public	2	5,6	**GENDER**	Woman	21	58,3
		Energy	1	2,8		Man	15	41,7
		Construction / Architecture	2	5,6		Total	36	100,0
		Total	36	100,0				

Assistant Managers and 15 Managers contributed to the study with their ideas. The homogeneous distribution of lower, middle and senior managers provides an advantage in order to have an overview of all areas of HRM.

When the distribution of the participants in terms of gender is examined, it is remarkable that the rates are close to each other. 58.3 % of them are women and 41.7 % are men. At one point, it would not be wrong to say that the range is not very clear, reducing the possibility of the study being uniform in terms of perspectives.

When the Fig. 1 above is examined, HRM Professionals have perceptually developed various responses and concerns when they first encountered the COVID-19 process. The most prominent of these is the feeling of "panic" expressed by 19 participants. In general, it would not be wrong to say that this is an expected result. Supplementarily, as stated in the previous dimension, 14 people stated that they were worried about "Unexpected Process." Similarly, 15 people underlined that they were uneasy due to "Uncertainty." With the start of the COVID-19 process, HRM Professionals suddenly find themselves in a situation that the modern business world has never encountered before, and the fact that a similar process has not been experienced before has shocked the participants in the managerial context before the crisis management and risk planning. Some of the participants explained this shock situation with statements such as "I stared at the wall for 1 hour and did not know what to do," "We returned to the fish out

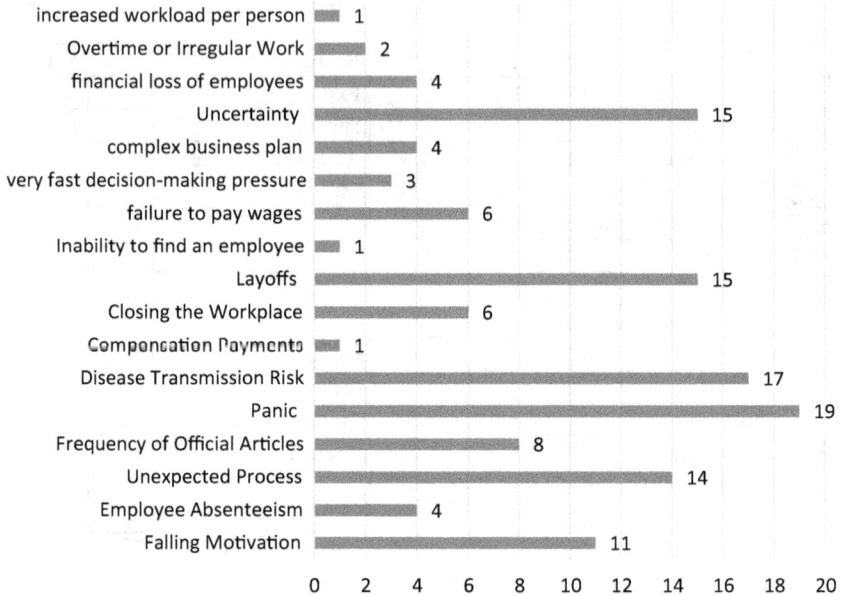

Fig. 1. HRM professionals' first reactions/ concerns about the process

of water." After the first shock wave, health concerns arose, which was reflected in the results of the study. 17 people expressed "Contamination Risk" as a cause for concern. With the detection of employees who test positive for COVID in some of the institutions of the participants, an atmosphere of "hysteria-sized panic" was blown within the institution as the participant stated. As a general judgment, the rate of concern increased among the participants, as it is not clear how to behave in business processes, although there is anxiety for those who work as human beings in the event of the spread or illness. In fact, one participant said, "Will COVID be considered a work disease? How will we carry out the compensation processes" and has entered an "uncertain" process in his own way. In the anecdotes quoted, since HR units had difficulty in controlling the panic atmosphere at the first stage, employees could not get satisfactory answers on issues such as occupational health safety, job security, material losses and continuity of wages. This situation has led to resignations, uneasiness and absenteeism. As can be seen in the Fig. 1 in all the elements related to this cause and effect relationship, this has created a concern for HRM professionals. Although the task of dismissal is mostly annoying, it has become more boring for HRM professionals during this process, with expressions such as "if they are dismissed they will not find a job again," "they are offended by the industry and they are destroyed" and "I am stuck between conscience and work" 15 participants were worried about the "Dismissals" that they had intensely anticipated. The confusion continues until the process of seeking a solution after the first panic wave mentioned above; as the number, variety and content of official articles on the process increase, HRM professionals start to get confused and have difficulty in decision-making, which means "frequency of official letters" with 8 people, "very fast decision making pressure" with 3 people, "complex business plan" with 4 people has emerged as anxiety. Some businesses have switched to unpaid leave, short-term allowance and similar practices, while others have switched to infrequent, alternating or online / home-working models. Participants expressed that there was a significant increase in the workload per person in this process. It emerges as one of the concerns in this regard. "Too much or Irregular Overtime" has been one of the concerns of HRM professionals regarding the compensation of falling productivity.

When the Fig. 2 above is analyzed, it is seen that HRM functions, which are at the center of the concerns of HRM professionals, are concentrated in two functions. These are "Wage Management" and "Recruitment" functions with 14 repetitions. As expected, HRM Professionals, who foresee that they will have difficulties in paying wages as a result of the crisis that may occur in the

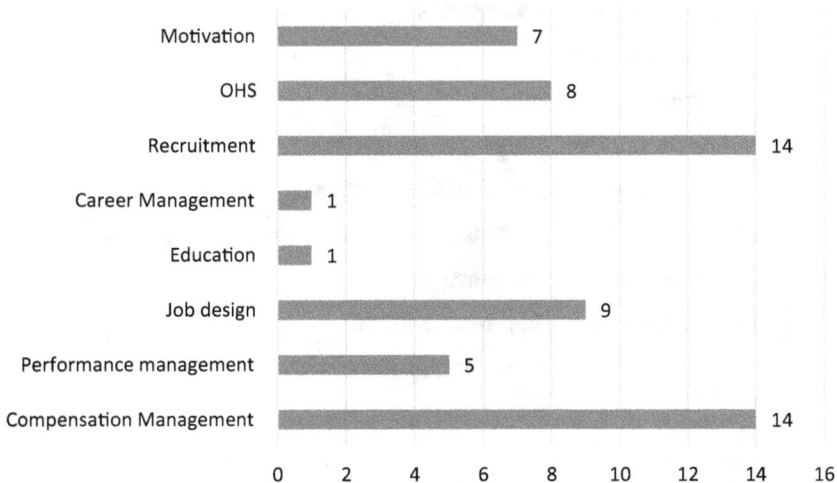

Fig. 2. HRM function that participants see in the center of concern

first stage, are intensely worried about the payments. Processes that may be encountered such as dismissal and unpaid leave and the anxiety of not meeting the employee's needs also brought the "recruitment" function to the fore. The fact that they could not locate COVID-19 until information came from the authorities at the beginning of the process confused whether this disease was an occupational disease status or a standard health problem. However, since it is unclear which enterprises will be revised under which conditions, when, what and which occupational health and safety procedures, they have become an issue of concern and entered the list. There are two more remarkable elements in expressions. First, for organizations that are not familiar with the online / home working method, evaluating employee performance and creating business plans suitable for this new transformation has put pressure on HRM professionals. Another factor is the "motivation" function, which has been ignored for many years or its disregard for its own expressions such as "I thought motivation consisted of a good library book" started to change during the COVID-19 process. Because factors such as uncertainties within the organization, risk of job security, and morale have created an atmosphere of tension and conflict. When the Organization began to be severely affected by the low motivation of the employees, they became concerned.

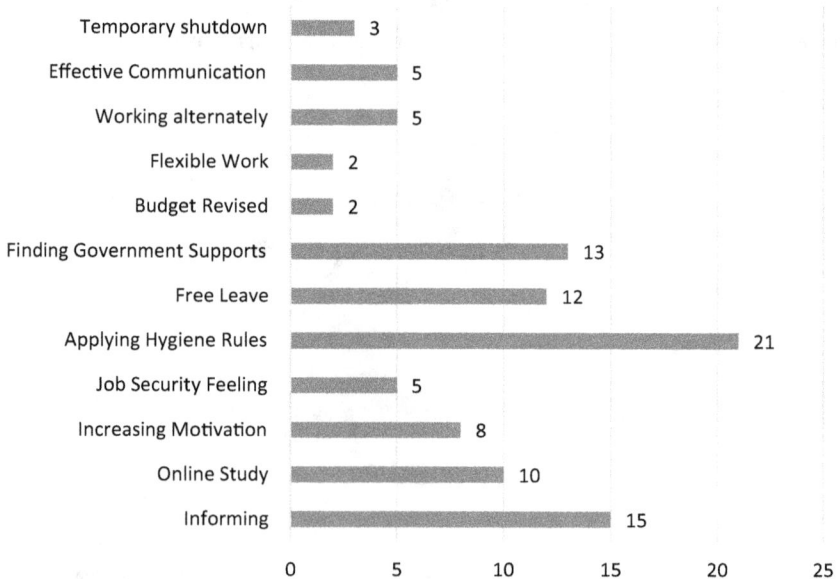

Fig. 3. First response methods preferences of HR professionals for the COVID-19 process

When the Fig. 3 above is examined, it is seen that HRM professionals prefer first intervention methods for the COVID-19 process. Parallel to the anxiety factors, 21 of the participants carried out the "enforcement of hygiene rules" intervention as a preliminary. Underlying this idea is the effort to improve health conditions and prevent the risk of transmission. The "informing" intervention was seen as another preliminary intervention by 15 people to dissipate the tense atmosphere of uncertainty and anxiety within the organization and to help the employees understand what to do. Preventing the loss of motivation in employees, which was also prominent in the previous Figure, is essential for organizations. For this reason, HRM professionals have tried to prevent employees from breaking their moral ties with the organization and to support the process in the continuation of practices such as "Increasing Motivation" methods, establishing "Effective communication" and creating "Job Security Trust." In the process, some organizations preferred the practice of "Temporary Workplace Closure" and preferred to follow the process (Later, there was state intervention in some sectors). Some have attempted to discover, seek and earn "state support" because their own crisis methods were insufficient to survive. Organizations continuing their working process have continued to serve by choosing different methods according to their business structures. Some organizations gave the right to work online / from home, especially to white and gold-collar employees who do not work directly on the production line. At this point, it was noticed that the opinions of HR professionals diverged.

While some of them profited the transformation positively, some did not lean towards efficiency. Different explanations, rather than the transformation to technology or innovation, underlie this concern. Some of these ideas "are not aware that they will put more strain on their backs," "you are not in control of working from home". "You are more controlled. You must be logged in to the VPN. From there, you are highly requested to enter daily efforts. So working from home is no fun. Because home is the place to rest. We designed our house for this. There are no areas and opportunities required by job security. Plus, the network quota you spend, heating, water, electricity and food belongs to you." "No break concept, you are constantly connected to the computer." Another criticism of online work is that, as the effect of sharing an emotional culture, the online work is mutually virtualizing organization and employee, and difficulties begin to emerge in emotion and empathy. Another criticism of online work is that, as the effect of sharing an emotional culture, the online work organization and the business are mutually virtualizing, and difficulties begin to emerge in emotion and empathy. One participant expresses this as "if they fire someone, that person is a little emoji for you." In the light of these concerns, different strategies were determined. One of them is "working in turns." Unlike the shift system, it appears as a hybrid model; certain days of the week online / from home, certain days of the week physically at the workplace. In this way, the lack of key personnel is prevented. Another model is "flexible working," in this working model, the employee can complete the weekly workload from home on a project-based context by deducting from working hours. As Uysal et al. (2020) mentioned in their studies, as the elderly population increases, death / case rates increase. Employees in key positions in companies are usually middle aged and older employees with experience. Therefore, protecting their health will also benefit the strategic sustainability of the organization. For this reason, HRM professionals have tried to keep middle aged and older employees in the system with the hybrid methods mentioned above.

When Fig. 4 is examined, the striking element is that the majority of the participants have the perception that the "Hygiene Rules" standards are revised again and that many practices will be permanent. Then again, from the similar theme, "Physical Distance" perception is established. Some participants even used the expressions "The biggest benefit of COVID-19 is that we finally get personal space" and "the torment of handshake is over." The code "Revising Business Plans / Models" is one of the most frequently featured ideas. Some organizations have had the opportunity to experience new business models

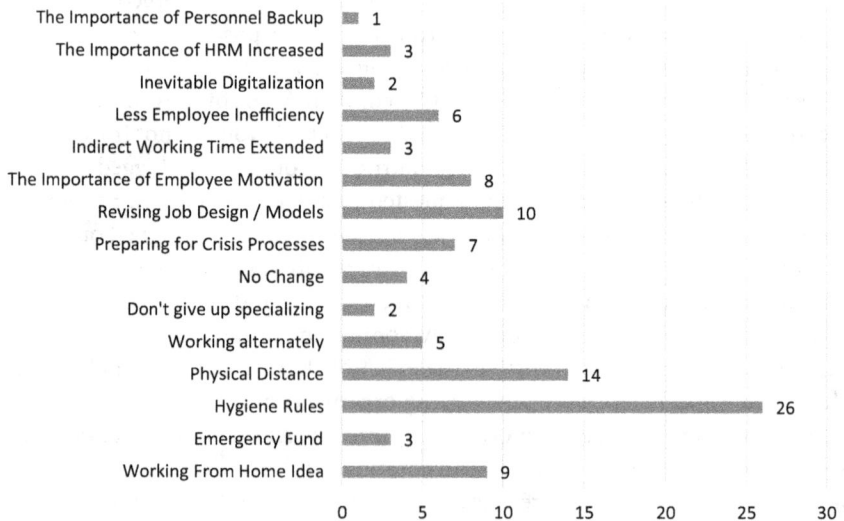

Category	Value
The Importance of Personnel Backup	1
The Importance of HRM Increased	3
Inevitable Digitalization	2
Less Employee Inefficiency	6
Indirect Working Time Extended	3
The Importance of Employee Motivation	8
Revising Job Design / Models	10
Preparing for Crisis Processes	7
No Change	4
Don't give up specializing	2
Working alternately	5
Physical Distance	14
Hygiene Rules	26
Emergency Fund	3
Working From Home Idea	9

Fig. 4. Perceptions of participants on the impact of the COVID-19 process on HRM

such as online / At Home / Take turns / Flexible, and those who are successful in this area express their intention to continue. As one participant stated, "Employee Motivation is not a myth" is one of the prominent ideas among HRM professionals, as justified in detail in previous chapters. In a process where business models are revised, new working orders are created, and the importance of motivation is rediscovered, "Understanding the importance of HRM" appears to be an inevitable result, albeit 3 times.

While struggling with some organizations for unpaid leave of absence, employee absenteeism, and resignation, the importance of "Employee Substitution" has come to the fore again. One participant expressed this situation as "what you said will never happen, what you said will never go is gone." This situation caused a chain reaction; The dream of achieving efficiency with fewer employees has turned into a complete fiasco with the change of HRM staff, and the indirect workload of the remaining employees has increased enormously. The reason for this is, in a way, over-specialization and business models consisting of employees who cannot substitute each other in the same unit. Another factor that emerged interestingly during the COVID-19 process is that "the harms of over-specialization" has emerged and understood. HRM staff had such difficulties financially in this process that they had to turn to all resources that could be found. Although it is an unexpected and unpredictable crisis, creating an "emergency fund" and preparing realistic "crisis plans" has emerged with the proactive aspects of HRM professionals.

4. Discussion

With the tension, fear and anxiety brought by uncertainty, black clouds started to circulate within the organization during the COVID-19 process. Over time, HRM became routine and predictable, but irreversibly transformed by the shock of COVID-19. In face of the unprecedented challenges that the COVID-19 crisis has imposed on businesses. Consequently, HR leaders have been forced to navigate unexplored waters, regardless of the industry they are in. However, the leaders of the Human Resources (HR) function have become the primary guardians of the health, safety, and well-being of employees (Vazquez and Puron, 2020).

While HRM professionals and experts thought that modern HRM was prepared for every situation and crisis, and its operations were in the process of routinization, they suddenly came face-to-face with an unknown unknown. In this case, both HRM professionals and researchers had to deal with the most classical HRM functions again. Working models called utopic or postmodern had to be tried and some of them were successful, while one of them completely resulted in a fiasco. With the COVID-19 process, there is a fact that is understood once again that it is almost directly or indirectly reflected in all participant responses, that HRM is still an indispensable department for organizations. Crises are often thought to be overcome with financial support only, but this process has shown that difficulties cannot be overcome without employee motivation and a properly designed working model.

Online / home working models had the opportunity to be tested during the application process. Even organizations that would never approach under normal conditions have experienced this practice. When cultural variables and local perceptions were involved, the results were sometimes not as expected. Employees who welcomed the application with excitement and happiness started to be disturbed over time. The basis of this is being constantly available, overtime, personal time-work time confusion. After this process, the system was revised in the presence of HRM professionals, and hybrid models more suitable for the culture were developed. In the infrastructure of these hybrid models, there is a desire not to break the organization-employee bond.

In this study, the preliminary perceptions and perspectives of HRM professionals regarding the COVID-19 process were examined. The study offers the opportunity to encounter perceptions and re-evaluate the reflections of the practices for future studies. In future studies, the reflections of the proposed hybrid models within entropy and the perspectives of HRM professionals after getting used to the crisis can be examined.

References

Akıncı, Z. (2011). Konaklama İşletmelerinde Kriz Sürecinde İnsan Kaynakları Yönetiminin Rolü ve Önemi, Suleyman Demirel University. The Journal of Visionary, 3(4): 132–152.

Allen, T. D., Cho, E., and Meier, L. L. (2014). Work–Family Boundary Dynamics. Annual Review of Organizational Psychology and Organizational Behavior, 1(1): 99–121.

Ata, I. (2020). How the COVID-19 Crisis Has Made HR One of the Most Important Jobs Today, https://www.entrepreneur.com/article/350747, Date of Access: 01.09.2020.

Atasoy, Y. (2020). Koronavirüs Salgın Sürecinde Evden Çalışma Modelinin Değerlendirilmesi, https://cdn.istanbul.edu.tr/FileHandler2.ashx?f=by_evdencalisma_ya.pdf, Date of Access: 03.09.2020.

Bingham, S. (2020). How HR Leaders Can Adapt to Uncertain Times, https://hbr.org/2020/08/how-hr-leaders-can-adapt-to-uncertain-times, Date of Access: 10.09.2020.

Crawford, F. (2020). The Post-COVID "New Normal" Workplace Has a Bright Future, https://www.sympli.com.au/blog/the-post-covid-new-normal-workplace-has-a-bright-future/, Date of Access: 10.09.2020.

Demirkıran, M., Taşkaya, S., and Dinç, M. (2016). A Study on the Relationship between Organizational Justice and Organizational Citizenship Behavior in Hospitals. International Journal of Business Management and Economic Research (IJBMER), 7(2): 547–554.

Gibson, C. B., and Gibbs, J. L. (2006). Unpacking the Concept of Virtuality: The Effects of Geographic Dispersion, Electronic Dependence, Dynamic Structure, and National Diversity on Team Innovation. Administrative Science Quarterly, 51(3): 451–495.

Grech, V. (2020). Unknown Unknowns–COVID-19 and Potential Global Mortality. Early Human Development, 144: 1–6, https://doi.org/10.1016/j.earlhumdev.2020.105026.

HBS. (2020). COVID-19 and the Workplace: Implications, Issues, and Insights for Future Research and Action, Harvard Business School, https://www.hbs.edu/faculty/Publication%20Files/20-127_6164cbfd-37a2-489e-8bd2-c252cc7abb87.pdf, Date of Access: 01.09.2020.

Huang, W. W., Wei, K. K., Watson, R. T., and Tan, B. C. Y. (2002). Supporting Virtual Team-Building with a GSS: An Empirical Investigation. Decision Support Systems, 34: 359–367.

Kane, R. L. (1998). Downsizing and HRM Strategy: Is There a Relationship?. International Journal of Employment Studies, 6(2): 43–69.

Kayhan Kuzgun, İ. (2007). Evde Parça Başı Ücret Karşılığı Çalışmada Bir Örnek Olay: Çivril'de Mum İşi, Yücel Pub., Ankara.

Lewis, N. (2020). HR Managers Rethink Their Role During the Coronavirus Pandemic, https://www.shrm.org/hr-today/news/hr-news/pages/hr-managers-rethink-their-work-coronavirus-pandemic.aspx, Date of Access: 10.09.2020.

Lositska, T. and Bieliaieva, N. (2020). Hr Crisis Management at Trade Enterprises. Eureka: Social and Humanities, 2020(1): 10–15.

Miles, M, B. and Huberman, A. M. (1994). Qualitative Data Analysis: An Expanded Sourcebook (2nd ed). Thousand Oaks, CA: Sage.

Moncrief, M. and O'Keefe, H. (2020). Houston HR Leaders Share Tactics and Strategies During Covid-19 Crisis, https://www.egonzehnder.com/functions/human-resources/insights/houston-hr-leaders-share-tactics-and-strategies-during-covid-19-crisis, Date of Access: 10.09.2020.

Özlü, A. and Öztaş, D. (2020). Yeni Corona Pandemisi (Covid-19) İle Mücadelede Geçmişten Ders Çıkartmak, Ankara Med Journal, (2): 468–481.

Şen, E. and Batı, G. F. (2020). COVID-19 Pandemik Krizinin Yönetim ve Ekonomi Politik Üzerine Olası Etkileri, Yönetim, Ekonomi ve Pazarlama Araştırmaları Journal, 4(2): 71–84.

Şimşek, M. Ş. and Aydoğan, E. (2000). Kriz Ortamlarında Stratejik İnsan Kaynakları Yönetimi Stratejisi, İktisadi ve İdari Bilimler, 14(1): 115–127.

TÜBA.(2020). Covid-19 Pandemi Değerlendirme Raporu, Türkiye Bilimler Akademisi Yayınları, TÜBA Raports No: 34, Ankara.

Uysal, B., Demirkıran, M., and Yorulmaz, M. (2020). Assessing of Factors Effecting COVID-19 Mortality Rate on a Global Basis, Turkish Studies, 15(4): 1185–1192.

Vazquez, C. and Puron, A. (2020). How HR Leaders Are Dealing with the COVID-19 Crisis A Digital Gathering with Top HR Leaders in Mexico, https://www.egonzehnder.com/functions/human-resources/insights/how-hr-leaders-are-dealing-with-the-covid-19-crisis, Date of Access: 10.09.2020.

Weggemans, G. and Bennick-Bai, X. (2020a). Leading with Care, Purpose, and Resolve during a Pandemic How HR Leaders Can Help Employees and Companies Weather the Coronavirus Crisis, https://www.egonzehnder.com/functions/human-resources/insights/leading-with-care-purpose-and-resolve-during-a-pandemic, Date of Access: 10.09.2020.

Weggemans, G. and Bennick-Bai, X. (2020b). HR Leadership Lessons from the Early Days of the COVID-19 Pandemic How Leaders Rapidly Readied Their Organizations and the Function to Respond to the Crisis and What Is to Come, https://www.egonzehnder.com/functions/human-resources/insights/hr-leadership-lessons-from-the-early-days-of-the-covid-19-pandemic, Date of Access: 10.09.2020.

Weisaeth, L., Knudsen, O., and Tomessen, A. (2002). Technological Disasters, Crisis Management and Leadership Stress. Journal of Hazardous Materials, 93(1): 33–45.

Yıldırım, A. and Şimşek, H. (2013). Sosyal Bilimlerde Nitel Araştırma Yöntemleri, Seçkin Pub., Ankara.

Yükseler, Z. (2020). Koronavirüs (Covid-19) Salgınının İstihdam ve Büyümeye Etkisi, https://zaferyukseler.academia.edu/research#papers, Date of Access: 02.09.2020.

Asst. Prof. Mehmet Dinç

The Effects of Stable Personalities and Situation-Specific Tendencies on Physical Distancing during the COVID-19 Pandemic: A Research on Organization Employees

1. Introduction

While the debate on the effects of information communication technologies (ICT) and Industry 4.0 on the workforce and employment continues, the COVID-19 pandemic that erupted in Wuhan, China, has led to a radical change in the private and public lives of people around the world (Ahrendt & Mascherini, 2020) and popularized the terms called "social distance" first and after a short time "physical distance" (Pratomo, 2020). Physical distance is used to mean that a person makes changes in their daily routines (avoiding crowded and unnecessary communities in a way that minimizes close contact with others, avoids joint meetings, reduces contact with people in higher risk groups such as the elderly and individuals with poor health) (The Canadian Agency for Public Health, 2020).

According to some researchers (Twardawski et al., 2020), physical distance refers to solidarity to protect others as an act of increasing social welfare and creates personal costs rather than personal benefits. They also defined physical distance as a means of obligation and rule-compliance, and argued that physical distance could be the subject of individuals' trust in authorities and their general willingness to comply with government rules. However, the adoption of these practices that reduce the spread of the virus by the country's governments, especially physical distance, and strict adherence to the proposed restrictions by the citizens did not occur at the same rate.

Based on this reality, it became important to develop an understanding of why some individuals are more willing than others to comply with such policies and measures that will reduce the spread of the pandemic (such as following physical distance behavior, wearing masks and isolating oneself at home). At this point, Miguel (2020) stated that there are large differences between individuals in the behavior of complying the containment measures against the pandemic, and Abdelrahman (2020) suggested that this difference is linked to psychological factors such as personality traits. Zettler et al., (2020) emphasized that the

Paradoxical Personality Consistency Theory (Caspi & Moffit, 1993) emphasizes the view that the differences in individuals' reactions to the COVID-19 pandemic are especially pronounced in changing and uncertain situations.

When the related literature is examined, it is seen that the following two groups of individual differences are suggested that can affect whether individuals comply with physical distance and other restrictions: Stable personality traits and situation-specific tendencies arising from the perception of pandemic conditions (Twardewski, Steindorf & Thelmann, 2020; Zajenkowski et al., 2020). For example, Twardawski et al., (2020) proposed three structures: anxiety, prosociality, and compliance with rules in individuals' adaptation to physical distance. They collected data from a large number of participants (N – 1.504) among German adult individuals. Theoretically, they examined the pandemic trends (beliefs and evaluations) and fixed personality traits (Neuroticism, Honesty-Humility (H) and Conscientiousness (C), representing the three sub-dimensions of the HEXACO model) related to these three structures in relation to the physical distance behavior reported by people and the motives they attach importance to. These researchers claimed that physical distance is a prosocial act and is related to the Honesty-Humility dimension as the basic personality structure, and also suggested a positive relationship between Conscientiousness and physical distance as the basic personality structure. For differences in people's solidary concern for others' is captured in the Honesty-Humility dimension and differences in orderliness and self-discipline are captured in the Conscientiousness dimension (Lee & Ashton, 2008). Zajenkowski et al., (2020) examined the role of personality traits (Big Five and Dark Triad) and perception of the COVID-19 pandemic situation (duty, intellect, mating, sociality, etc.) in explaining individual differences in compliance with government restrictions in Poland.

During the COVID-19 pandemic, studies that found that compliance with principles, adoption of these principles and reaction to the determined restrictions were predictors of many personality traits took place in the literature. For example, in a Qatar study (N = 405) conscientiousness and neuroticism individuals showed more tendency to practice physical distance behavior to avoid transmission of COVID-19 (Abdelrahman, 20202). In the previously published US study (N = 501) examining the psychosocial and other patterns of compliance with the COVID-19 principles (10 principles), individuals with particularly conscientiousness traits reported greater compliance in the 7-day period (Bogg & Milad, 2020).

In another study (N = 502), conscientiousness and agreeableness traits predicted the promotion of physical distance and hygiene, receiving general public health messages (Blagov, 2020). In a large-scale Brazilian study (N = 715), they further considered the need for individuals with low extroversion and high conscientiousness to avoid approaching people (physical distance) until the COVID-19 situation is under control. (Carvalho, Pianowski & Gonçalves, 2020). In a study involving participants from 22 countries (N = 996), it was found that individuals with high conscientiousness traits participated in stockpiling more toilet paper, but the Honesty-Humility personality was not a significant predictor of toilet paper stocpiling (Garbe, Rau & Toppe, 2020).

In a study conducted on the basis of two separate samples (N = 200 and N = 401) in the United Kingdom, it was found that Honesty-Humility personality trait predicted past and future hoarding avoidance behavior (Columbus, 2020). In a German study, most of which were made up of individuals with prosocial tendencies (N = 419), people stated that they used preventive measures primarily to protect themselves and secondly to bring the people to a protective value. Preventive measures such as physical distance and hand washing have been the subject of communication as effective ways to protect the self and the public (Leder, Pastukhov & Schütz, 2020). Investigating the role of individual differences in the pandemic in nine personality traits and 17 COVID-19 criteria in five independent samples from two Western European countries (overall N = 10,702), Zettler et al. (2020) found that personality traits, including prosocial and collaborative tendencies, are consistent predictors of behavioral regulation. He found that H trait showed consistent relationships in relation to physical distance, hygiene, and advice.

This study is based on Twardewski et al. (2020)'s work in the context of Germany. But making small changes in Turkey's three provinces located in the Western Mediterranean Region (Antalya, Isparta and Burdur) was preceded to adapt sampling. Therefore, this study focus on two aims. The first objective is to determine the effect of the Honesty/ Humility and Conscientiousness (2 of the factors that make up the HEXACO model of personality) traits of these working individuals on their physical distancing behavior. The second objective is to determine the effect of self-protection and social welfare motives perceived by working individuals, their beliefs about other people's physical distancing, and their trust in and acceptance of authorities (situation-specific tendencies) on their physical distancing behavior. By collecting data employee individuals who work in the public and private sectors, to achieve this goal, the following hypotheses can be proposed based on the above study findings:

H_1: *Honesty-Humility personality trait of the organization employees has a significant and positive effect on their physical distance behavior.*

H_2: *Conscientiousness personality trait of the organization employees has a significant and positive effect on their physical distance behavior.*

H_3: *Beliefs of the employees of the organization in the physical distance behaviors of other people have a significant and positive effect on their physical distance behavior.*

H_4: *The self-protection and social welfare motives of the organization employees have a significant and positive effect on their physical distance behavior.*

H_5: *The trust of the employees of the organization in the authorities and their tendency to adopt them have a significant and positive effect on their physical distance behavior.*

2. Methods

This section will include information about the purpose and the model of the research, the universe and sample of the research, and the scales used in the study.

In this study, two objectives were aimed by examining the stable personality differences in physical distancing behaviors of adult individuals working in the public and private sectors during the COVID-19 period and the differences in their tendencies specific to the situation (COVID-19 pandemic). The research model designed in this context is presented in Figs. 1 and 2.

The study sample consists of individuals eighteen years of age and older, working in the public and private organizations, located in the cities Antalya,

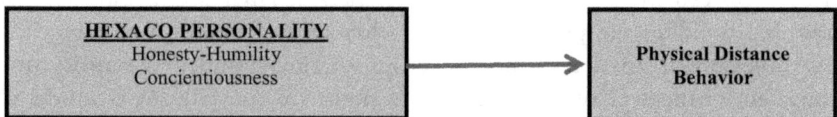

Fig. 1. First model of research

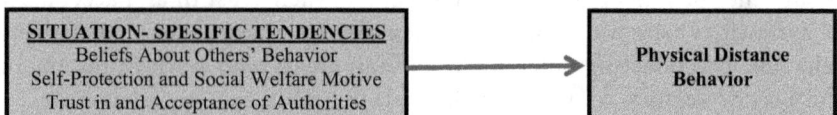

Fig. 2. Second model of research

Isparta, and Burdur, in the Western Mediterranean Region of Turkey. Inclusion criteria are being an active employee and being qualified as an adult. In this context, a survey was conducted in line with the permission obtained from the Turkish Ministry of Health and then from the Ethics Committee of the State University, of which the researcher is a staff member, as the subject of the study is the COVID-19 Pandemic. Data collection was carried out online, via Google Forms. The link of the questionnaire was shared via social media (Facebook) and WhatsApp Messenger application; Individuals were invited to participate and the snowball strategy was preferred to reach more participants. A total of 581 people from three provinces participated in the study by answering the questions in the questionnaire. As a result of the examinations of the question-naire forms, it was determined that some of them had missing data enough to exclude them from the analysis. In some forms, it was determined that the participants did not actively work in a public or private sector organization. In total, 110 forms were excluded from the analysis. Analyses were carried out using the data obtained from a total of 471 valid questionnaires.

When the public and private sector employees that make up the sample were examined, it was determined that 56.5 % were women, 61.8 % were married, 46.5 % were undergraduates, 31.2 % had a master's degree, and 77.5 % lived in a city center. 54.8 % of the participants were employed in the public and 45.2 % in the private sector. The age of the employees varied between 18 and 62, with an average age of 35.28 (SD = 11.17).

This research was carried out using a questionnaire with 6 parts. In the sixth part of the form, there are 6 questions asked in order to determine the demographic characteristics of the employees. In the other 5 parts of the ques-tionnaire form, there are statements regarding the variables used in the study. Detailed information about the scales is presented below.

The Brief HEXACO Personality Inventory: In the Brief HEXACO Personality Inventory, Honesty/Humility and Conscientiousness traits are considered as independent variables. The HEXACO Personality Inventory was first devel-oped by Lee and Ashton (2004) and has a long form consisting of 100 items and a short form consisting of 60 items. The brief form used in this study was developed by de Vries (2013). The scale, which consists of 6 dimensions and 24 items, is a 5-point Likert type questionnaire. The scale is evaluated as 1: Completely Disagree and 5: Completely Agree. In the study, Honesty/Humility and Conscientiousness traits were measured with four items for each personality trait in this brief form developed by de Vries (2013) mentioned above. In the Honesty/Humility trait, 3 items are coded in reverse, while in the Conscientiousness trait, 2 items are coded in reverse. 8 statements that measure these two personality traits were retrieved from Dinç and Akçakanat's (2020) study and used in this research. The statements "*I have difficulty lying (Honesty/Humility)*" and "*I work very carefully (Conscientiousness)*" can be given as examples.

Physical Distancing Scale: This scale constitutes the dependent variable of the research. It was developed by Twardawski, Steindorf, and Thielmann (2020) and consists of 6 items and one dimension. The scale was developed by the researchers to show the extent to which participants participated in physical distancing during the COVID-19 Pandemic. While developing the scale, the researchers focused on the implemented behaviors based on the recommendations by the Robert-Koch Institute to slow the spread of the virus. In the scale, all items are answered on 6-point Likert scales ranging from 1 = Completely Disagree to 6 = Completely Agree. There is a reverse-scored item in the scale. Physical Distancing Scale was translated into Turkish by the researcher and used in this study. The phrase "*I avoided close greeting rituals (such as hugging, handshaking)*" can be given as an example.

Trust in and Acceptance of Authorities Scale: This scale, which represents the first of the situation-specific tendencies of the employees in the study and used as an independent variable, was developed by Twardawski, Steindorf, and Thielmann (2020) and consists of 4 items and one dimension. The researchers developed this scale to reveal the extent to which participants trusted their government's actions to slow the spread of the COVID-19 Pandemic and to what extent they followed the rules set by them. The 6-point Likert type scale, translated into Turkish by the researcher, is evaluated as 1: Completely Disagree and 6: Completely Agree. There are no reverse-scored items on the scale. The statement "*I trust the measures taken by the government to slow the spread of the Coronavirus*" can be given as an example.

Beliefs About Others' Behavior Scale: This scale, which represents the second of the situation-specific tendencies of the employees in the study and used as another independent variable, was developed by Twardawski, Steindorf, and Thielmann (2020) and consists of 6 items and one dimension. When the researchers developed this scale, they used the same list as the participants' own physical distancing and asked the participants to rate their beliefs about others' engagement in physical distancing. The 6-point Likert type scale, translated into Turkish by the researcher, is evaluated as 1: Completely Disagree and 6: Completely Agree. There are no reverse-scored items on the scale. The statement "*People in my social circle tried to stay away from others as much as possible whenever they left their homes.*" can be given as an example.

Self-Protection and Social Welfare Motive Scale: This scale represents the third of the situation-specific tendencies in the study and used as another independent variable. Originally, the scale was developed by Twardawski, Steindorf, and Thielmann (2020) in order to show the motives (such as protecting oneself and relatives, protecting the welfare of the society) of participating in all physical distancing behaviors reported by the participants in order to measure the motives for physical distancing. The 6-point Likert type scale, translated into Turkish by the researcher, is evaluated as 1: Completely Disagree and 6: Completely Agree. There are no reverse-scored items on the scale. The statement *"In order to protect the society in which I live (my citizens in general), I tried to stay away from others whenever I left my house."* can be given as an example.

SPSS 22 and AMOS 21 were used for the analysis of the research data. Descriptive statistics were used to reveal the demographic characteristics of the participants in the study. In the study, confirmatory factor analysis was also used to test the validity of the scales used; Internal consistency coefficient methods were preferred to test the reliability. Pearson's correlation analysis was used to analyze the relationships between the 5 variables used in the study. Multiple regression analysis was used to determine the effect of stable personality traits and situational tendencies on physical distancing.

3. Results

The findings obtained as a result of the data analysis are presented below.

3.1. Validity and Reliability Analysis of the Scales

Structural validity was examined to test the validity of the scales used in the study. Confirmatory factor analysis was used to reveal the construct validity since all scales were previously tested and validated for different cultures. AMOS software was used for analysis and the highest predictability method was chosen. In this context, the goodness of fit values obtained as a result of the confirmatory factor analysis are presented in Tab. 1.

As can be seen in Tab. 1, the goodness of fit values of the 6 scales used in the study are within acceptable limits. These values show that the scales are structurally valid. In all scales, modifications were made in scale items without discarding them. As a result of the analyses, the one-dimensional structures of the six scales preferred in the study were preserved as they were in the original studies.

Tab. 1. Goodness of fit values of scales

Variables	χ²/df	CFI	NFI	GFI	AGFI	RMSEA
Honesty-Humility	3,97	.97	.96	.99	.95	.080
Conscientiousness	2.31	.97	.95	.92	.89	0.70
Trust in and Acceptance of Authorities	3.66	.99	.99	.99	.96	0.75
Beliefs about Others' Behavior	2.94	.99	.98	.98	.95	0.35
Self-Prot. and Soc.	4.81	.96	.95	.92	.87	0.90
Welfare Motive Physical Distance	1.58	.99	.98	.99	.97	0.35
Acceptable Fit*	≤5	>0.90	>0.90	>0.85	>0.80	<0.08
Good Fit	≤3	>0.97	>0.95	>0.90	>0.85	<0.05

*Joreskog ve Sorbom, (1993); Kline, (1998); Anderson ve Gerbing, (1984).

Tab. 2. Internal consistency coefficients of the scales

Variables	Item Number	α	Skewness	Kurtosis
Honesty-Humility	4	.71	-.320	.208
Conscientiousness	4	.76	-.217	-.431
Trust in and Acceptance of Authorities	4	.80	-.532	-.040
Beliefs about Others' Behavior	6	.89	-.481	-.047
Self-Protection and Social Welfare Motive	12	.95	-.577	-.602
Physical Distance	6	.82	-.882	.248

Internal consistency (Cronbach's Alpha) coefficients were calculated to test the reliability of the scales. The coefficients calculated for the scales are presented in Tab. 2.

As can be seen in Tab. 2, for all variables used in the study, coefficients were calculated as above .70, which is the generally accepted limit in the literature (Nunnally, 1978). In light of all this information, it can be stated that all scales are structurally valid and reliable. In Tab. 2, before proceeding with the hypothesis tests, it was also investigated whether the data showed a normal distribution or not. As a result of the analysis made by examining the skewness/kurtosis coefficients, it was found that the skewness and kurtosis coefficients were within the range of ±1, as suggested by Morgan et al. (2004: 49). Based on this result, parametric techniques were used in the research.

Tab. 3. Betimsel istatistikler ve değişkenler arasi ilişkiler

Variables	Mean.	S.D.	1	2	3	4	5	6
1. Honesty-Humility	3.39	.69	(.71)					
2. Conscientiousness	4.00	.54	. 182**	(.76)				
3. Trust in and Acceptance of Authorities	4.17	1.11	.161**	.061	(.80)			
4. Beliefs about Others' Behavior	4.51	.88	.019	.085	.029	(.89)		
5. Self-Protection and Social Welfare Motive	5.42	.54	.078	.274**	.123**	.273**	(.95)	
6. Physical Distance	5.37	.57	.147**	.243**	.072	.285**	.769**	(.82)

** p< .01, values in parentheses indicate the reliability coefficients of the dimensions, N= 471

3.2. Findings Regarding the Relationships between Variables

Pearson's correlation analysis was conducted to reveal the relationships between the independent and dependent variables. Tab. 3 presents the arithmetic mean and standard deviation values of the variables as well as the correlation coefficients.

As can be seen from Tab. 3, the social distancing level of the employees participating in the study during the COVID-19 Pandemic is relatively high with an arithmetic average of 5.37 (SD = .57). When the tendencies of the participants specific to the COVID-19 Pandemic situation are examined, Self-protection and Social Welfare Motive levels are the highest with an arithmetic mean of 5.42 (SD = .54), Beliefs About Others' Behavior levels are high with an arithmetic average of 4.51 (SD = .88) and Trust in and Acceptance of Authorities levels are 4.17 (SD = 1.11), which still can be called fairly high.

When the participants are evaluated in terms of two dimensions of the HEXACO Personality Model, it is seen that they consider themselves Conscientiousness people with an arithmetic average of 4.00 (SD = .54). Again, it is determined from Tab. 3 that Honesty / Humility (Mean = 3.39, SD = .69) personality trait observed in the participants is above average.

When the correlation analysis results in Tab. 3 are examined, it is determined that there is a positive correlation at a high power level (r = .769, p <.01) between Self-protection and Social Welfare Motive, one of the trends specific to the COVID-19 Pandemic situation, and physical distancing. It was determined that there is a significant positive relationship between Beliefs

About Others' Behavior, another trend specific to the situation, and physical distancing, at a low-power level (r = .285, p <.01). No significant relationship was found between Trust in and Acceptance of Authorities and physical distancing.

Considering the relationships between the two dimensions of the HEXACO Personality Model and Physical Distancing, it was determined that there is a significant relationship between the Honesty/Humility and Conscientiousness dimensions and Physical Distancing. In this context, positive and low-power level, significant relationships were found between the Conscientiousness trait and Physical Distancing (r = .243, p <.01) and between the Honesty/Humility trait and Physical Distancing (r = .117, p <.01).

When the relationships between the two dimensions of the HEXACO Personality Model and the situation-specific tendencies were examined, a positive and low-strength relationship was found only between the Honesty/ Humility personality trait and Trust in and Acceptance of Authorities (r = .147, p <.01). A positive and significant relationship at low-power level was found only between the Conscientiousness trait and Self-protection and Social Welfare Motive (r = .274, p <.01).

3.3. Findings Regarding Hypothesis Tests

With the help of regression analysis, the analysis made for the hypotheses of the research will be explained with the help of tables in the next part of the study. Multiple linear regression analysis was used to test the hypotheses. The Enter method, which is one of the frequently used methods was preferred in variable selection. In this context, firstly, it was checked whether the necessary assumptions were met in order to perform multiple linear regression analysis. The Durbin-Watson coefficient being between 1.5 and 2.5 and the Variance Inflation Factor (VIF) coefficients being less than 10 show that there are no autocorrelation and multiple connection problems (Büyüköztürk, 2013). The Durbin-Watson coefficient in this study ranged between .932 and 1.380; VIF values were in the range of 1.015–1.096. Accordingly, no autocorrelation or multicollinearity problems were observed. Before proceeding to the regression analysis, the distribution of the data was examined and the skewness and kurtosis coefficients were examined for this purpose. According to Tabachnick and Fidell (2012), the skewness and kurtosis coefficients being between −1 and +1 indicate that the data are distributed normally. As a result of the analysis, it was determined that the kurtosis coefficients were between −0.602 and 0.248, and the skewness coefficients between −0.882 and −0.217. In light of these values,

Tab. 4. Results of multiple regression analysis for the effect of stable personality traits as physical distance behavior dependent variable

Independent Variables	β	t	p
Honesty-Humility	0,106	2,332	0,020
Conscientiousness	0,223	4,924	0,000
R²=0,070 Adj. R²=0,066 F=17,524 (p=0,000)			

it was observed that the data fit the normal distribution. As a result, it can be stated that the regression model established is linear.

In this part of the study, firstly, in light of the First Model, the analysis results regarding the effects of the independent variables Honesty/Humility and Conscientiousness personality traits on the dependent variable, the physical distance behaviors, will be presented. Then, in accordance with the Second Model, the area of the focus will be the analysis results regarding the effect of the independent variables Trust in and Acceptance of Authorities, Beliefs About Others' Behavior, and Self-protection and Social Welfare Motive on physical distancing.

Tab. 4 contains the results of the regression analysis presenting the effects of Honesty/Humility and Conscientiousness personality traits on Physical Distancing of public and private sector employees. As seen in Tab. 4, the regression model yielded significant results ($F = 17.524$; $p < 0.05$). The adjusted R^2 value, which is the proportion of the variance for the dependent variable (Physical Distancing) that's explained by the independent variables (Honesty/Humility and Conscientiousness), was calculated as 0.070. This result shows that 7.0 % variance in Physical Distancing is explained by the Honesty/Humility and the Conscientiousness traits. When the Beta coefficients in the table are examined, it can be seen that both variables produced significant effects in explaining Physical Distancing when both independent variables were put in the regression model. Among the independent variables in the regression model, Honesty/Humility reveals a significant effect as $β = -0.106$, $p = 0.020$, and Conscientiousness $β = 0.223$, $p = 0.000$. Therefore, it can be stated that the H1 and H2 hypotheses suggested in the study are supported.

Tab. 5 shows the results of the regression analysis presenting the effect of Trust in and Acceptance of Authorities, Beliefs About Others' Behavior and Self-protection and Social Welfare Motive on Physical Distancing of public and private sector employees. As can be understood from Tab. 5, the regression

Tab. 5. Results of multiple regression analysis for the effect of situation- specific tendencies as physical distance behavior dependent variable

Independent Variables	β	t	p
Trust in and Acceptance of Authorities	-0,023	-0,766	0,444
Beliefs about Others' Behavior	0,081	2,657	0,008
Self-Protection and Social Welfare Motive	0,750	24,415	0,000
R^2=0,598 Adj. R^2=0,596 F=231,721 (p=0,000)			

model yielded statistically significant results (F = 231.721; p <0.05). The adjusted R^2 value, which is the proportion of the variance for the dependent variable (Physical Distancing) that's explained by the independent variables (Trust in and Acceptance of Authorities, Beliefs About Others' Behavior, and Self-protection and Social Welfare Motive), was calculated as 0.598. This result shows that the 59.8 % variance in Physical Distancing is explained by Trust in and Acceptance of Authorities, Beliefs About Others' Behavior, Self-protection, and Social Welfare Motive. When the Beta coefficients in the table are examined, it can be seen that two variables (Beliefs About Others' Behavior – Self-protection and Social Welfare Motive) produced significant effects in explaining Physical Distancing when all three independent variables were included in the regression model. However, one variable (Trust in and Acceptance of Authorities) did not produce significant effects. Among the independent variables in the regression model, Beliefs About Others' Behavior reveals a significant effect as $β = -0.081$, p = 0.008, and Self-protection and Social Welfare Motive as $β = 0.750$ p = 0.000. However, one of the independent variables in the regression model, Trust in and Acceptance of Authorities Tendency, did not reveal a significant effect ($β = -0.023$; p = 0.444). Therefore, it can be stated that the H3 and H4 hypotheses suggested in the study are supported, but the H5 hypothesis is not.

4. Discussion

In the first half of 2020, the pandemic caused by the coronavirus disease 2019 (COVID-19) and still maintaining its contagious and lethal effect especially with age-related variables such as life expectancy at birth (Uysal, Demirkıran & Yorulmaz, 2020), created an unexpected situation for people. Policies and efforts implemented to reduce the spread and contagious effect of the COVID-19 virus made people feel under an existential threat, restricting their freedom in their individual and business lives. In this process, many measures such as physical distance and hand hygiene were recommended by WHO. However, issues such as how individuals react to the these measures and the changing situations of COVID-19, what factors increase and decrease individuals' levels of compliance with precautions, attracted the attention of social and behavioral scientists. While physical distance efforts aim to eradicate the virus and improve public health, this has also fueled interest as they pose unforeseen challenges to all public or private organizations and their employees. This study examines the stable personality traits (Honesty-Humility and Conscientiousness) and also pandemic-specific tendencies (trust in and acceptance of authorities, beliefs about others' physical distancing, self- protection and social welfare).

As a result of the analyzes carried out, the first and second hypotheses of the study were supported. According to the results of the analysis conducted to test the first hypothesis of the study within the scope of the first model, a significant and positive effect of the Honesty-Humility personality trait on physical distance behavior was determined. In other words, as the public and private sector employees got higher scores in the Honesty-Humility trait, they paid more attention to physical distance behavior, which is preventive behavior against pandemics. This finding obtained from the study is consistent with the results of many studies (Twardewski et al., 2020; Zettler et al., 2020) that pro-vide correlative evidence that Honesty-Humility personality trait increases compliance with preventive health behaviors that reduce pandemics in general and physical distance behaviors in particular.

Again, the analysis results made to test the second hypothesis of the study in accordance with Model 1 revealed that the Conscientiousness personality trait significantly and positively affected the physical distance behavior, as ex-pected. More specifically, employees experienced an increase in their physical distance behavior as the Conscientiousness trait improved. This finding was consistent with the results of many studies. That is, among the general charac-teristics of individuals with Conscientiousness is confidence and self-reliance in overcoming barriers to compliance (Bogg & Milad, 2020). Compliance with rules reflects the prototype of this personality, Conscientiousness individuals are successful in following socially defined norms and delaying gratification when necessary (Roberts et al., 2009). These personality-dominant individuals further considered the need to avoid approaching people until the Coronavirus situation is under control (Carvalho et al., 2020).

While the third and fourth hypotheses of the study proposed under the Model 2 were supported, the fifth hypothesis was not. According to the results of the analysis conducted to test the third hypothesis of the study, the beliefs of the employees of the organization in the physical distance behaviors of other people had a significant and positive effect on their physical distance behavior. This finding coincided with the results of many previous studies. For example, Twardawski et al. (2020) stated that individuals' cooperation in social dilemmas such as a pandemic will be greater if they believe that other people around the actors will also cooperate. Thus, they suggested that the physical distance behavior of individuals may show strong positive relationships with beliefs about other people's participation in this behavior. Zajenkowski et al., (2020) found that belief about whether other people conform to physical distance behavior positively affects an individual's compliance with physical distance behavior as a situation specific disposition. Bogg and Milad (2020) found that people who perceive people around them as supportive of behaviors such as physical distance or encouraging them to follow these rules will follow these rules more.

According to the results of the analysis conducted to test the fourth hypothesis of the study, it was revealed that the self-protection and social welfare motives of the organization employees had a significant and positive effect on their physical distance behavior. This finding supported the results of several studies conducted in the literature. For example, Leder et al., (2020), in the study that most of the participants consisted of individuals with prosocial tendency, stated that the participants used protective measures against COVID-19 primarily to protect themselves, secondly to bring the public to protective value, and also preventive measures such as physical distance to self and They found that they were the subject of communication as an effective tool to protect the public. Twardawski et al., (2020) found that physical distance behavior in the physical distance relationship with H is focused on the social welfare motive. Columbus (2020) also revealed a similar motive for stockpiling behavior in the COVID-19 process.

According to the results of the analysis conducted to test the fifth hypothesis of the study, it was found that the organization employees' trust in and acceptance of authorities did not have a significant effect on their physical distance behavior. This finding was not consistent with the study findings of Twardawski et al., (2020) and Zajenkowski et al., (2020) on which the study was based. The researchers stated that trust in political institutions and adoption of the rules set by the authorities will reinforce obedience in society and positively affect physical distance.

Theoretically, the findings of this study provide an opportunity for a better understanding of the responses of these employees to the pandemic through their physical distance behaviors during the pandemic process, based on the fixed personality characteristics of public and private sector employees and their specific tendencies to the pandemic situation. In the course of the COVID-19 pandemic, the direction of the organization's employees' behavior can only be predicted if their stable and situation-specific tendencies are known. In addition, this study presents reflections on the factors that predict the adoption of adaptive or precautionary behaviors in particular physical distance in order to avoid transmission during the pandemic process.

The study has some limitations. First, this study is based on a cross-sectional research design that evaluates participants' perceptions on a particular subject within only one time frame. Second, the measurement tools preferred for the research are based on self-reporting, the researcher cannot be included in the answers, and thus the participants only report their personal perceptions instead of the measured structure itself. Third, the relationships between variables examined in the study are only within a single culture and cover certain provinces. So we can not generalize the results of the public and private sector employees in the whole of Turkey represents another limitation. Fourth, the effect of Emotionality, eXtraversion, Agreeableness and Openess to Experience personality traits in the HEXACO model on physical distance behavior was not examined in this study.

References

Abdelrahman, M. (2020). Personality traits, risk perception, and protective behaviors of Arab residents of Qatar during the COVID-19 pandemic. International Journal of Mental Health and Addiction. https://doi.org/10.1007/s11469-020-00352-7

Ahrendt, D., & Mascherini, M. (2020). Living, working and COVID-19. Eurofound First Findings Report – April 2020.

Anderson, J. C., & Gerbing, D. W. (1984). The effect of sampling error on convergence, improper solutions, and goodness-of-fit indices for maximum likelihood confirmatory factor analysis. Psychometrika, 49(2), 155–173.

Blagov, P. S. (2020, March 28). Adaptive and dark personality traits in the Covid-19 pandemic: Predicting health-behavior endorsement and the appeal of public-health messages. https://doi.org/10.31234/osf.io/chgkn

Bogg, T., & Milad, E. (2020, April 3). Slowing the spread of COVID-19: Demographic, personality, and social cognition predictors of guideline adherence in a representative U.S. sample. https://doi.org/10.31234/osf.io/yc2gq

Brouard, S., Vasilopoulos, P., & Becher, M. (2020). Sociodemographic and psychological correlates of compliance with the COVID-19 public health measures in France. Canadian Journal of Political Science, 53, 253–258. https://doi.org/10.1017/S0008423920000335

Büyüköztürk, Ş. (2013). Sosyal bilimler için veri analizi el kitabı. Ankara: Pegem Akademi.

Carvalho, L. de F., Pianowski, G., & Gonçalves, A. P. (2020). Personality differences and COVID-19: Are extroversion and conscientiousness personality traits associated with engagement with containment measures? Trends in Psychiatry and Psychotherapy. https://doi.org/10.1590/2237-6089-2020-0029

Caspi, A., & Moffitt, T. F. (1993). When do individual differences matter? A paradoxical theory of personality coherence. Psychological Inquiry, 4, 247–271.

Columbus, S. (2020). Who hoards? Honesty-humility and behavioural responses to the 2019/20 coronavirus pandemic. https://doi.org/10.31234/osf.io/8e62v

De Vries, R. E. (2013). The 24-item brief HEXACO inventory (BHI). Journal of Research in Personality, 47(6), 871–880.

Dinç, M., & Akçakanat, T. (2020). The mediating role of proactive personality in the relationship between HEXACO personality and motivation to learn: A study on hospitality sector employees. In: Şule Aydın, Bekir Bora Dedeoğlu & Ömer Çoban (Eds.), Organizational behavior challenges in the tourism industry. IGI Global, pp. 387–410. ISBN:9781799814900, DOI: 10.4018/978-1-7998-1474-0.ch021

Garbe, L., Rau, R., & Toppe, T. (2020). Influence of perceived threat of Covid-19 and HEXACO personality traits on toilet paper stockpiling. https://doi.org/10.31219/osf.io/eyur7

Jöreskog, K., & Sörbom, D. (1993). LISREL 8: Structural equation modeling with the SIMPLIS command language. Chicago, IL: Scientific Software International Inc.

Kline, R. B. (1998). Principles and practice of structural equation modeling. New York: Guilford Press.

Leder, J., Pastukhov, A., & Schütz, A. (2020, March 30). Even prosocially oriented individuals save themselves first: Social value orientation, subjective effectiveness and the usage of protective measures during the COVID-19 pandemic in Germany. https://doi.org/10.31234/osf.io/nugcr

Lee, K., & Ashton, M. C. (2004). Psychometric properties of the HEXACO personality inventory. Multivariate Behavioral Research, 39(2), 329–358.

Miguel, F. K., Machado, G. M., Pianowski, G., & Carvalho, L. F. (2020). Compliance with containment measures to the COVID-19 pandemic over time: Do antisocial traits matter?. Personality and Individual Differences, 168(2021), 110346. https://doi.org/10.1016/j.paid.2020.110346

Morgan, G. A., Leech, N. L., Gloeckner, G. W., & Barret, K. C. (2004). SPSS for introductory statistics: Use and interpretation. Second Edition. London: Lawrence Erlbaum Associates.

Nunnally, J. C. (1978). Psychometric theory. Second edition. New York: McGraw-Hill.

Pratomo, H. (2020). From social distance to physical distance: A challenge for evaluating public health interventions against COVID-19. Kesmas (National Public Health Journal), 15(2). http://dx.doi.org/10.21109/kesmas.v15i2.4010

Roberts, B. W., Jackson, J. J., Fayard, J. V., & Edmonds, G. (2020). Conscientiousness. In: Leary, M. & Hoyle, R. (Eds.), Handbook of individual differences in social behavior. New York, NY: Guilford, pp. 369–381.

Tabachnick, B. G., & Fidell, L. S. (2012). Using multivariate statistics. Sixth edition. Boston, MA: Allyn and Bacon.

The Canadian Agency for Public Health. Physical distancing: Actions for reducing the spread of Covid-19. 2020 April 15 [cited 2020 May 3]. Available from: https://www.canada.ca/en/publichealth/service/publications/diseasesconditions/physical-distancing.html.

Twardawski, M., Steindorf, L., & Thielmann, I. (2020). Three pillars of physical distancing: Anxiety, prosociality, and rule compliance during the COVID-19 pandemic. PsyArXiv. July 16. doi:10.31234/osf.io/zkfyb.

Uysal, B., Demirkıran, M., & Yorulmaz, M. (2020). Assessing of factors effecting COVID-19 mortality rate on a global basis. Turkish Studies, 15(4), 1185–1192. https://dx.doi.org/10.7827/TurkishStudies.44390

Zajenkowski, M., Jonason, P. K., Leniarska, M., & Kozakiewicz, Z. (2020). Who complies with the restrictions to reduce the spread of COVID-19? Personality and perceptions of the COVID-19 situation. Personality and Individual Differences, 166, Article 110199. https://doi.org/10.1016/j.paid.2020.110199.

Zettler, I., Schild, C., Lilleholt, L., & Böhm, R. (2020). Individual differences in accepting personal restrictions to fight the COVID-19 pandemic: Results from a Danish adult sample. https://doi.org/10.31234/osf.io/pkm2a

PhD. Elvan Öztürk

Investigation of COVID-19's Effects on Financial Markets and Economy

1. Introduction and Literature Review

The COVID-19 epidemic that occurred in Wuhan, China's Hubei province towards the end of 2019, spread rapidly around the world, it has required that the epidemic be qualified as a pandemic by the World Health Organization. On December 29, 2019, 4 cases were reported, all linked to the Huanan (South China) Seafood Wholesale Market (Li et al., 2020). Wuhan Municipal Health Commission, China, reported a cluster of cases of pneumonia in Wuhan, Hubei Province. A novel coronavirus was eventually identified (WHO, 2020). The first case outside of China was reported by the authorities on January 13, 2020, and after that date, the number of cases started to increase all over the world, showing a rapid acceleration. After the World Health Organization announced that the virus was transmitted from human to human on January 21, 2020, with the number of cases reaching 118.319 worldwide on March 11, 2020, WHO stated that this rapid increase can be described as a pandemic. On the same day it was announced by the Ministry of Health's first cases seen in Turkey. Following the first case, there have been limitations extending to the present day due to the fact that it is stated to be short term but the increase in the number of cases continues and it is a threat that affects public health. In this process, educational institutions from primary school to university have suspended face-to-face education and the distance education system has become widespread. All kinds of artistic, scientific and cultural activities have been postponed; The services of places where citizens may be in close contact such as restaurants, hairdressers and recreational areas have been stopped or regulated. The number of cases has also been tried to be controlled with restrictions such as curfews and long-distance transportation being subject to permission. As can be seen from the Graph 1, the number of cases, which started to increase rapidly starting from the day the first case was seen, decreased in a period of 2 months as a result of the restrictions.

Although the measures taken to prevent the pandemic from spreading have an improving effect on public health, this pandemic also has an economic dimension. Namely, the process is inevitable that affect the not only Turkey

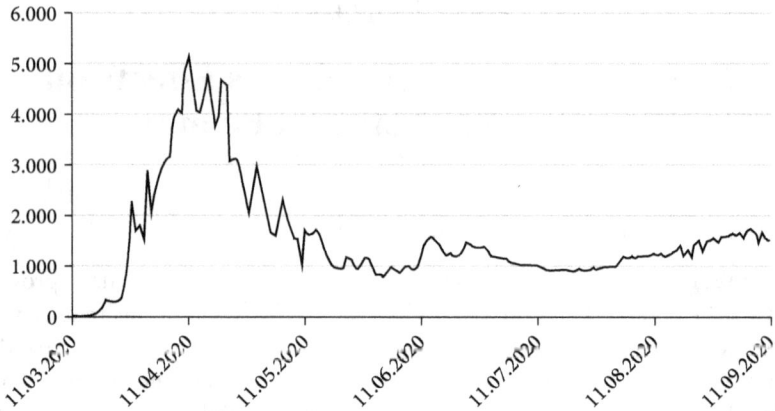

Graph 1. Number of patients (per day). **Source:** It was created with data from the official website of the Ministry of Health (MoH, 2020)

but also entire world economy. As a result of the start and spread of the pandemic in China, the economic life in the country has come to a halt, production has shrunk, and China, whose economic growth is largely dependent on exports, has faced a serious economic crisis because other countries have stopped their imports with China for fear of further exposure to the virus. As it is the second largest economy in the world, the economic changes in China affected almost the whole world in succession. According to Bloom et al. (2020), the slowdown of the Chinese economy with production cuts also interrupted the functioning of global supply chains. Firms around the world, regardless of their size, started to experience contractions in production due to inputs from China. This result can be understood more clearly when looking at traditional trade networks.

In the Fig. 1, the size of the bubble states the size of the country (worth of trade) and the thickness of the linking lines states the relative significance of bilateral flows. Looking at the traditional trade networks of China in all goods and services, it is seen how important it is in world trade. China is truly the world's workshop, at the center of the entire global network. Therefore, the production cut in china will create secondary supply shocks in manufacturing sectors in almost all countries (Baldwin and Mauro, 2020; 15). In the figure, it is understood that in Turkey compared to other countries do more trade with China. Therefore, to clarify the situation in Turkey, it is possible to see through

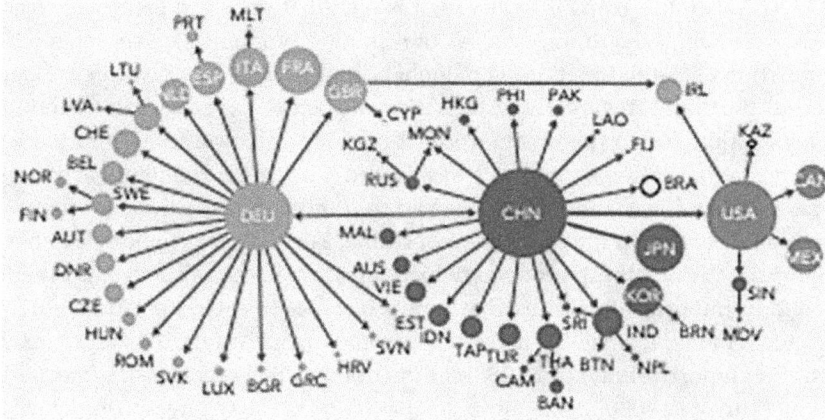

Fig. 1. Traditional trade networks (all goods and services). **Source:** Li et al. (2019)

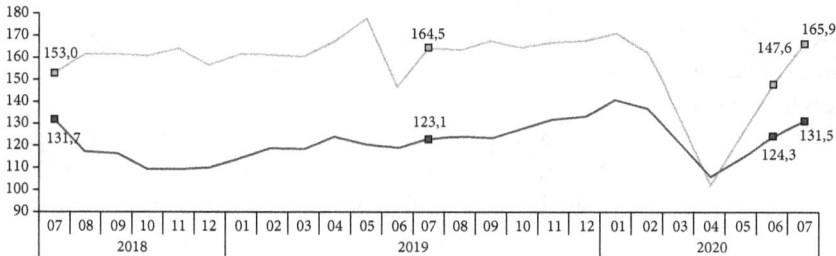

Graph 2. Seasonal and calendar adjusted foreign trade volume indices, July 2020 (2010=100). **Source:** Turkish Statistical Institute Foreign Trade Indices (Turkstat, 2020a)

changes as of the date on tables or graphs. According to data published by Turkey's Statistics Institute shows changes in foreign trade indices.

The value at the top with a value of 153.0 in the graph gives the export value, and the value below, starting with 131.7, gives the import values. Looking at the seasonal and calendar adjusted foreign trade quantity indices dated July 2020, it is observed that the import and export indices started to decline, especially as of January 2020, when the pandemic started. The export volume index, which was 168.6 in December 2019, decreased by 39 % to 102.8 in April 2020, and the import volume index, which was 133.0, decreased to 102.3 with a decrease

Elvan Öztürk

of 23 %. When the graph is analyzed, it is seen that there is a greater decrease in exports compared to imports. As the Chinese economy slowed down with production cuts, the functioning of global supply chains was disrupted. Firms around the world, regardless of their size, started to experience contractions in production due to the inputs from China, The narrow and even forbidden transportation between countries has slowed worldwide economic activities. (McKibbin and Fernando, 2020). Referring to foreign trade indices, the contraction occurring in the production of China, Turkey seems to be able to have an impact. China's cheap products, which rank first in the world in exports and second in imports, are also used as inputs in other countries (Eğilmez, 2020). As shown in Fig. 1, when the dates range from January to July 2020 assessment, with the import volume of 12 288 million dollars, Turkey's largest importer is China (Turkstat, 2020b). Therefore, since it is one of the strongest trading partners, a trade crisis happening in China can also affect Turkey. Within the scope of the policies taken by the Ministry of Commerce regarding the COVID-19 pandemic, it was stated that on February 7, 2020, it was decided to temporarily stop the import of all kinds of live and non-living animals, animal products and by-products from China. The decision was repealed on 1 May 2020. The Ministry made the assessment that this situation will contribute to the process in our export of agricultural products (MoC, 2020). It is known that especially imports in foreign trade affect the industrial production index (Barışık and Yayar, 2012). Therefore, in order to make a more effective interpretation, it is necessary to look at the industrial production index as well as foreign trade data. "Industrial Production Index" is calculated in order to measure the positive or negative effects of the developments in the industrial sector of the economy and the applied economic policies in the short term (Turkstat, 2020c).

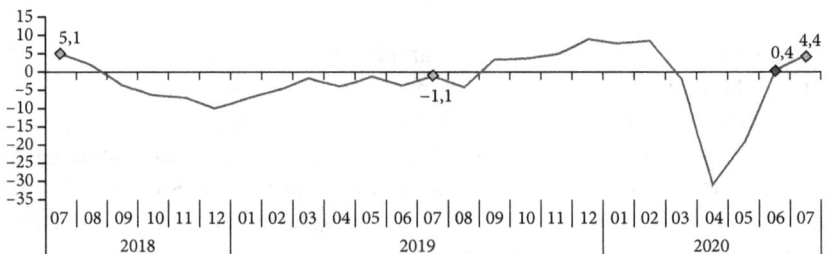

Graph 3. Industrial production index annual change rates (%), July 2020. **Source:** Turkish Statistical Institute Industrial Production Index (Turkstat, 2020c)

Similar to the seasonal and calendar adjusted foreign trade volume indices, a decrease occurred in the industrial production index from February 2020 to April 2020. Considering the change rates, it is seen that in April 2020, compared to the same month of the previous year, a change of – 49.3 % in durable consumption goods, – 42.9 % in capital goods and – 39.4 % in medium-high technology. In total, a decrease of 31.3 % is observed in April 2020 compared to the same month of the previous year. In the analysis conducted since January 2006, it is seen that the industrial production index has not changed at this level for about 14 years. This great change in the industrial production index is likely to directly affect economic growth. Likewise, it is known that the causality relationship between the industrial production index and economic growth is positive. This shows that the effect of an increase or decrease in the industrial production index on economic growth will be in the same direction. Based on this finding, it is understood that economic growth and industrial production feed each other and have a long-term relationship (Terzi and Oltulular, 2004). Economic growth represents the increase in the amount of final goods and services produced in a country in a given period. The concept of economic growth, which is an expression of the increase in real income per capita, basically defines long-term increases in production capacity that concern the supply side of the economy (Akiş, 2020: 7). When the literature is examined, it has been observed that the GDP (Gross Domestic Product) variable is generally taken as an indicator of economic growth (Grossman and Krueger, 1995; Jones et al., 1998; Oskooe, 2010).

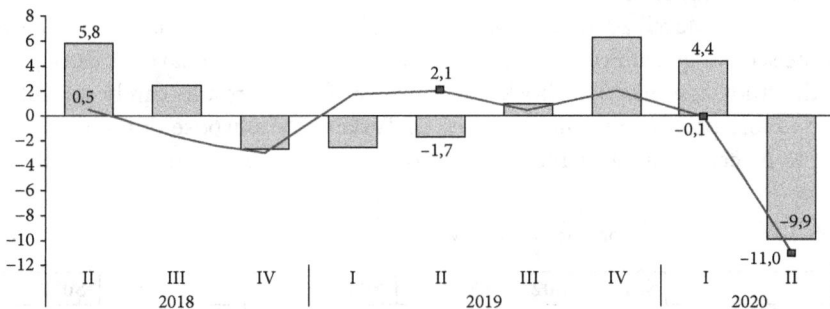

Graph 4. GDP growth rate (%), Quarter II: April-June, 2020. **Source:** Turkish Statistical Institute Quarterly Gross Domestic Product, Quarter II: April-June, 2020 (Turkstat, 2020d)

The columns in the figure show the change rate compared to the same quarter of the previous year, while the line shows the change rate compared to the previous quarter. In the second quarter of the year covering the April–June 2020 period, it is seen that there is a 9.9 % decrease compared to the same quarter of the previous year. In the same period, services, one of the branches of economic activity that affected the growth rate of GDP, represented the biggest decrease with 25 %. industry showed a decrease of 16.5 %, but financial and insurance activities showed the highest increase with 27.8 %. The serious decrease in foreign trade and industrial production causes the gross domestic product to decrease. The study of Mckibbin and Fernando (2020) shows that even an inclusive epidemic can significantly affect the global economy in the short term. They have explored seven different scenarios for how COVID-19 could evolve next year, by developing a global hybrid DSGE / CGE general equilibrium model to better understand possible economic consequences such as economic growth. In the study where they examine the macroeconomic results of different scenarios and their effects on financial markets, scenarios 1 through 3 (called SO1, SO2, and SO3) suppose epidemiological events are limited to China. Scenarios 4 and 6 (S04, S05 and S06) are pandemic scenarios in which epidemiological shocks happen to varying degrees in all countries. Scenarios 1 to 6 suppose that the shocks are temporary. For Scenario 7 (called S07), it is anticipated that a small pandemic will recur every year in an uncertain future. If COVID-19 turns into a global epidemic, the results show that the cost in lost economic output began to rise to trillions of dollars.

Pandemic scenarios (4,5 and 6th scenarios) indicate a GDP contraction of 5.5 % can be experienced in Turkey looking at the study Mckibbin and Fernando published in March 2020. However, when we look at the real data, a 9.9 % decline in the second quarter of 2020 is seen to occur in Turkey. Scenarios 1 through 6 in the study assumes that shocks are temporary, so the results can be expected to be more positive in other quarters in Turkey. The purpose of their work is not to be certain about pandemic, but rather to ensure information about the

Tab. 1. COVID-19 Scenarios for Turkey

	S01	S02	S03	S04	S05	S06	S07
% GDP loss	-0,1	-0,2	-0,2	-1,4	-3,2	-5,5	-1,2
GDP Loss in 2020 ($US billions)	-3	-4	-6	-33	-75	-130	-30

Source: Mckibbin ve Fernando (2020)

probable economic costs of the illness. Likewise, at the time this article was written on March 4, 2020, the possibility of any of these scenarios and the scope of reasonable alternatives are rather unclear. If COVID-19 turns into a global pandemic (WHO labeled the outbreak as a pandemic on March 11), the results of the study suggest that the cost could rise rapidly. The authors emphasize that a series of policy reaction will be required both in the short term and in the next years (Mckibbin and Fernando, 2020).

Measures taken for the control of the pandemic in Turkey in this process has brought to many businesses closing point. In an economic system operating in a cycle, breaking of one link of the chain may cause the other rings to break. As a matter of fact, employers who have to close their workplaces may need to dismiss their employees if they do not have reserve funds. Naturally, this process causes the employer, whose operation is closed, to suspend its financial relationship with its suppliers, and thus the trouble experienced by a single enterprise can spread to thousands of companies. In this process, the story of dismissal that started with a single business can turn into unemployed individuals who were fired from thousands of companies. Regarding this example, labor force statistics are included in the study. Changes in labor force data during the COVID-19 pandemic period are given in Graph 5.

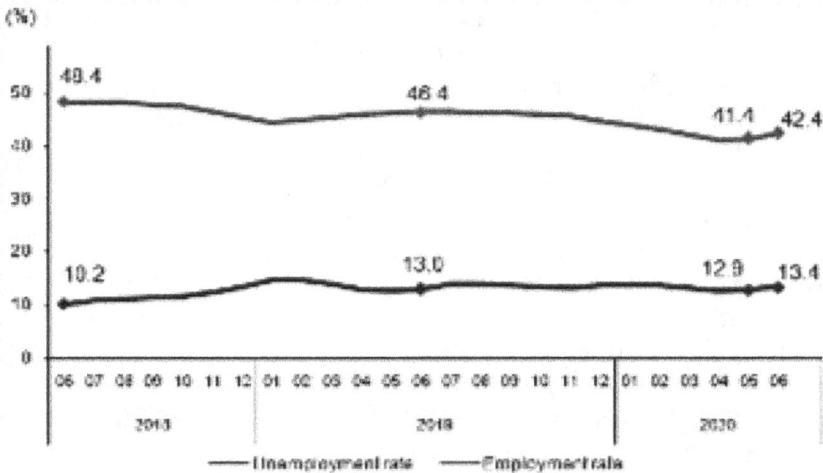

Graph 5. Unemployment and employment rate, June 2018-June 2020. **Source:** Turkish Statistical Institute Labour Force Statistics, June 2020 (Turkstat, 2020e)

The value at the top with 48.4 in the graph gives the employment rate, and the value below, starting with 10.2 gives the unemployment rate. Referring to the latest labor force statistics released on statistical values across Turkey shows that those children above the age of 15 and 13.4 % for the year, the unemployment rate in June 2020. Thus, by the standards of Turkey Statistical Institute, according to the previous month, 275,000 people remained unemployed. The relationship between employment and growth is interpreted as an increase in gross domestic product, which is an indicator of growth, to increase production and thus increase the demand for labor (Güçlüoğlu, 2017). The amount of goods and services produced and the labor demand decreases due to the decrease in real GDP in a country, the number of employed people decreases and unemployment increases in parallel (Ünsal, 2004; 12). It is possible to support this statement when the change in GDP and the course of unemployment rates are evaluated based on the data. Unemployment rates increase in the same period while the GDP data for the second quarter are trending downwards. Kasseh (2018) supports this data by stating that unemployment represents a significant waste of a country's manpower resources and therefore one of the most serious obstacles to economic progress.

Turkey has been forced to contend with high unemployment rates in nearly every period onwards the 1960s. Especially after the 1980s, unemployment, which started to increase due to globalization and technological progress, reached levels that are considered high compared to universal measures in the 1990s. With the 2001 crisis, the employment problem further became stronger, and the rescue after the crisis was very slow and limited, unlike the rescue in economic growth. Causes such as speedy population growth, problems in education policy, insufficient investment, political and economic instability caused this problem to become more severe (Ay, 2012; 322). High labor costs also have an increasing effect on unemployment (Onaran, 2002). In line with the measures taken during the pandemic process, businesses whose production / service has been suspended fall into financial difficulties because they cannot generate any income.

It is understood from the graphs that the relationship between economic growth and unemployment is in reverse as stated in the literature. Economic growth, unemployment and inflation are the biggest macroeconomic problems of our age. Inflation and unemployment are closely related concepts, especially in the short term. Attempts to decrease unemployment have often been accompanied by an rising in inflation, and attempts to decrease inflation often led to an rising in unemployment (Pal, 2018). The anxiety created by the pandemic forced the states to take some measures. It is inevitable that preventing the

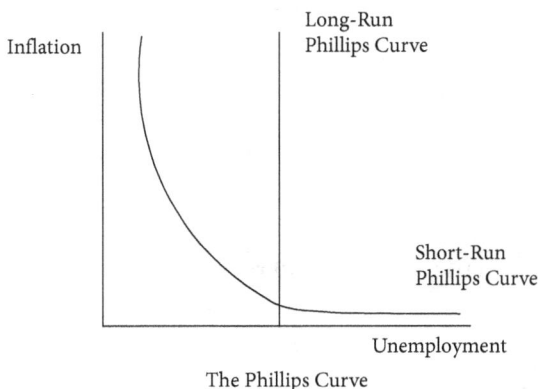

The Phillips Curve

Fig. 2. Phillips curve. **Source:** Alisa (2015)

increase in unemployment numbers with practices such as a dismissal ban will affect other macroeconomic indicators and financial markets. The relationship between inflation and unemployment, one of the most important macroeconomic indicators of countries, was first named as the Phillips curve by Phillips (1958) in the article titled "The Relation between Unemployment and the Rate of Change of Money Wage Rates in the United Kingdom, 1861–1957."

Phillips curve clearly shows that there is an inverse relationship between unemployment and inflation. The increase in unemployment in the short run causes a fall in inflation. Another statement for the Phillips curve is that it is easier for producers and workers to increase prices and wages during times of economic growth. High unemployment obligates employees to accept lower wages. Conversely, as we approach full employment, there is an increased demand for additional factors of production. The growth of total demand in the economy makes new unbalances and psychologically rises limited resources. Thus, the increase in inflation accelerates with the increase in demand (Phillips, 1958; Alisa, 2015). It is necessary to look at inflation data to observe the relationship between unemployment and inflation. When the unemployment rates given in Graph 5 are analyzed, it is seen that there has been an increase from April to June. Looking at the inflation rates, an increase was observed from April to June, but a decrease occurred afterwards.

When the graph is analyzed, inflation has also increased with the increase in unemployment in the same periods. However, it may not be possible to measure the effects of the pandemic in the short term. Supply chain disruptions in some

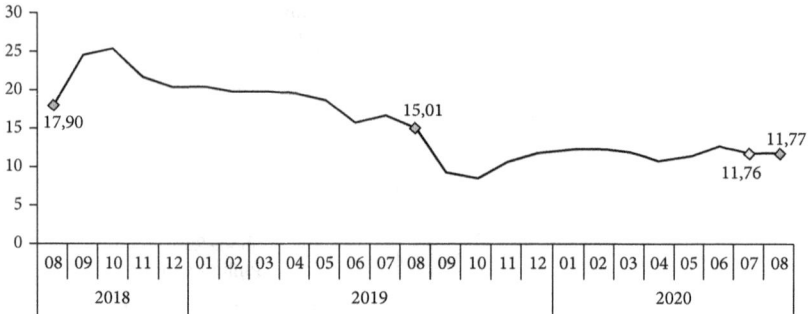

Graph 6. Annual rate of changes in Consumer Price Index (%), August 2020. **Source:** Turkish Statistical Institute Consumer Price Index, August 2020 (Turkstat, 2020 f)

countries can result in prolonged price increases, which could lead to higher inflation. At this point, governments must remain loyal to their inflation expectations with strong policies. One of the most important points for this is the fight against unemployment. Hiring subsidies can be an important component of financial strategy to encourage firms to hire unemployed individuals (IMF, 2020a).

Some measures have been taken to prevent the increase in unemployment during the pandemic. The prohibition of dismissal among the decisions taken in this process is one of the most important decisions in terms of its economic impact. With the provisional article added to the Labor Law numbered 4857 on April 16, 2020, the termination of all kinds of business or service contracts by the employer for 3 months is prohibited. Exceptions to this prohibition are situations and similar reasons that do not comply with the rules of ethics and goodwill, expiration of fixed-term business or service contracts, closure of the workplace for any reason and the termination of its activity, all kinds of service purchases made in accordance with the relevant legislation and termination of work in construction works. The employer may allocate the employee wholly or partially unpaid leave for a period not exceeding three months from the effective date of this law article. Providing unpaid leave to the employee within the scope of this law article does not give the employee the right to terminate the contract based on a just cause. In the application of the dismissal prohibition for 3 months, the period was extended until 17 November 2020, later. In addition, the President has the authority to extend these periods until 30 June 2021 (Resmi Gazete, 2003).

A monthly net wage of 1,168 TL is given to the employee who is taken on unpaid leave by the employer with the provisional article added to the Unemployment Insurance Law No. 4447 (Resmi Gazete, 2020). As of August 2020, the possibility of living with a wage of 1.168 Turkish Liras (TL) should be evaluated in the country where the hunger limit of a family of four is 2.384 TL, the poverty line is 7.765 TL(Türkiş, 2020) and the minimum wage is 2.324.70 TL. Likewise, even if the employee receives short-time work allowance, this amount will constitute 60 % of the daily average gross earnings calculated by taking into account the earnings subject to premium for the last twelve months (Resmi Gazete, 2011). In this process, it should be considered how an individual who balances her/his income expense and has debts will sustain her/his life as a result of a serious loss of income. As such, the individual will have to cut back their spending and will not want to spend except for their basic needs. As a matter of fact, an individual who cuts his expenditures cannot be expected to saving. In this way, the balance that is tried to be created in the economy by preventing unemployment will turn into an imbalance created by the individual who cuts consumption and savings because of loss of income. As a matter of fact, in the economic system operating in a cycle, the costs of companies that interrupt their production / services in line with the measures taken to prevent the spread of the pandemic will increase, and this will naturally be reflected in the prices of goods / services. With the increase in prices, the decrease in the demand of the individual, who has already reduced his expenditures to basic needs, may cause a serious recession in the economy. According to IMF (2020b), "pandemic risks sustain important. Pandemics could repeat in places that seem to have gone past peak infection, requiring the reimposition of at least some containment measures. A more long period decline in activities could cause to further scarring, including from wider firm closures. Financial circumstances may again squeeze as in January–March, displaying fragilities among borrowers. This could tip some economies into debt crises and slow activities further. Financial conditions may again tighten as in January–March, exposing vulnerabilities among borrowers. This could tip some economies into debt crises and slow activities further. More generally, cross-border spillovers from poorer external demand and tighter financial conditions could further enlarge the impact of country- or region-specific shocks on global growth. Beyond pandemic-related downside risks, escalating tensions between the United States and China on multiple fronts, battered relationships among the Organization of the Petroleum Exporting Countries (OPEC)+ coalition of oil producers, and widespread social restlessness pose additional challenges to the global economy. Moreover, against a ground of low

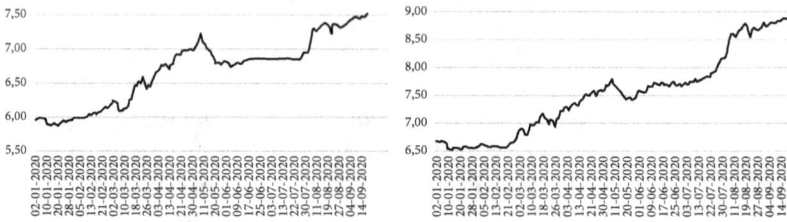

Graph 7. Exchange rate, USD/TRY and EUR/TRY (January, 2-September,14). **Source:** It was created with data from the official website of the CBRT (CBRT, 2020a)

inflation and high debt (particularly in advanced economies), protracted weak total demand could cause to further disinflation and debt service difficulties that, in turn, weigh further on activity."

Almost all businesses borrow money to keep their workflows and rely on the income they will earn to payoff that debt. If an unspecified shock like the COVID-19 process causes a sudden stop in income, the situation is expected to result in bankruptcy (Baldwin and Mauro, 2020; 18). While the pandemic causes loss of income and debt repayment problems in companies, income items such as declining exports and tourism may disrupt the balanced growth target and cause an increase in the current account deficit and pressure on the exchange rate. Liquidity squeeze in global markets will also emerge as another factor that will put pressure on the exchange rate. This will cause difficulties in fulfilling foreign currency liabilities. Repayments of foreign debt used by the private sector in financing large investments with the guarantorship of state banks are also at risk in this sense (Yorulmaz and Kaptan, 2020; 25). In Graph 7, Dollar / TRY and Euro / TRY exchange rates are given since the beginning of the year.

Looking at the exchange rates, a serious increase has been observed in the EUR / TRY parity since January 2020. The EUR / TRY parity, which was 6.67 on January 2, 2020, increased by 33 % on September 14, 2020 and became 8.88. Similarly, the USD / TRY parity has been in an upward trend since the beginning of the year with an increase of 27 %. Looking at the Central Bank of the Republic of Turkey data, there has been a 38 % decrease in foreign exchange reserves since the beginning of the year (CBRT, 2020b). Foreign exchange (FX) reserves play an important role in achieving macroeconomic policy targets and preventing possible financial crises in that they provide maneuvering space for the sustainability of the exchange rate regime and monetary policies (CBRT, 2020c). The decrease in foreign exchange reserves, which are also used as an intervention tool in the market, is a concern for investors both in the domestic and foreign markets.

A common crisis contagion vector in financial crises is the exchange rate. As an example, in the Asian crisis of the late 1990s, it affected companies and countries that borrowed in one currency and earned revenue in another. Examining the Thai case, many Thai companies went bankrupt because of the sudden exchange rate devaluation, the dollar value of their income could not meet the dollar interest cost and loan repayment obligations. (Baldwin and Mauro, 2020; 23). Considering the risk of the real sector in Turkey by the end of 2019, the domestic and external debt of the real sector a total of 2 trillion 600 billion 966 million Turkish Liras. Foreign currency debt constitutes 61 % of the total debt (CBRT, 2020d). Thus, the real sector entered 2020, when COVID-19 started, with a high foreign exchange debt and exchange rate risk. The CBRT (2020e) applied a "Survey of the Effects of the Pandemic on the Real Sector" between 31 March and 7 April. According to the results of the survey, it is seen that 28.8 % of the companies stopped production during the pandemic process. The most important problem faced by companies in this process has been re-ported as a decrease in orders. Increasing financing difficulties, logistics disruption, supply problems and cost increases are among the other problems related to the epidemic. Firms rated commercial bank credits as the most important tool for dealing with cash flow shortages. When asked which headings policies they think would be more effective in order to maintain pre-epidemic employ-ment level, "personnel expenses," "taxes" and "access to finance" were cited as the most important topics. The survey applied to manufacturing industry com-panies at the beginning of April presented a useful picture on the basis of sector and scale in order to determine the effects of COVID-19 on the real sector in a timely manner and to design appropriate policies. In this direction, the Ministry of Treasury and Finance stated that they have prepared an Economic Stability Shield Package supported by 100 Billion Lira. With this package, pre-serve employment, support the real sector and trades, and the pandemic might occur by controlling the impact on Turkey's economy is intended to reduce potential damage to a minimum. Some of these measures, especially covering companies, are as follows (PIO, 2020);

- Thus, it is possible for the employee, who is not dismissed due to the inter-ruption of work due to compulsory reasons, and whose wages continue to be paid, in addition to his own working hours for 4 months after the commence-ment of the work, on the condition of not exceeding the maximum daily working time of 11 hours.

- Short Work Allowance has been put into use. When the measures were announced, it was stated that the support would be until 31 August, but it was stated that the application would continue until 31 October by extending the time for 2 more months. In addition, 6 billion TL was transferred to approximately 4.5 million people with short-time work allowance, unemployment allowance and cash wage support.
- In the sectors of retail, iron and steel, automotive, logistics, transportation, cinema and theater, accommodation, catering, textile and event organization, the tax returns, VAT deductions and social security payments for April, May and June 2020 have been postponed by the decision.
- Loan principal and interest payments to banks of companies whose cash flow has deteriorated due to the measures related to the COVID-19 pandemic were postponed for a minimum of 3 months and additional financing support was provided when necessary. Within the scope of the Craftsmen Support Package, the state bank Halkbank provided 16 billion 906 million TL financial support to 684,103 tradesmen. Thus, the expenses of enterprises without income were tried to be postponed and layoffs were prevented.
- Accommodation tax application has been postponed until November. Thus, it is aimed to positively affect the tourism sector, which was heavily affected by the epidemic process.
- Easement fees and revenue share payments for hotel rentals have been postponed for 6 months for April, May and June.
- In domestic airline transportation, which has a VAT rate of 18 %, this rate has been reduced to 1 % for three months.
- During this period, the principal and interest payments of the loan debts to Halkbank, the state bank, of the tradesmen and craftsmen who declared that their business was negatively affected, were postponed for 3 months and without interest.
- Due to the COVID-19 process, companies that went into default in April, May and June were recorded as "force majeure" in their credit registers. Minimum wage support is continued.
- The Credit Guarantee Fund limit was increased from TRY 25 billion to TRY50 billion, and the priority in loans was given to companies and SMEs with liquidity needs and collateral deficits, as they were negatively affected by developments. The Credit Guarantee Fund allocated TRY 151 billion 734 million financing to 192,645 companies. 97 % of these companies are SMEs.
- The Central Bank postponed the principal and interest payments of the open rediscount loan for April, May and June to October, November and

December and the maximum maturity was extended by 1 year. The commitment closing periods of the rediscount credits that expired in April, May and June have been extended by 1 year.

- Appropriate and advantageous credit packages for citizens have been encouraged. For this reason, following the announcement of the package, state banks have offered individual customers with a monthly household income of TRY 5,000 or less, a loan with monthly equal installments up to TRY 10,000 with a 6-month grace period under the name of basic needs support package. In this context, TRY 39 billion 117 million was provided to 6 million 617 thousand citizens.
- It was stated that approximately 2 million families determined by the Ministry of Family, Labor and Social Policies will be given TRY 1,000 in cash support. This number has reached 5.5 million families.
- The mortgageable amount has been increased from 80 % to 90 % in houses below TRY 500 thousand, and the minimum down payment has been reduced to 10 %. In fact, mortgage loans with a maturity of up to 180 months and a grace period of up to 12 months were used in public banks. In fact, housing loans with a maturity of up to 180 months and a grace period of up to 12 months were used in public banks. Housing sales in August 2020 increased by 54.2 % compared to the same month of the previous year with the effect of these loans.

It has been stated that the Economic Stability Shield Package reached TRY 260 Billion in total until the end of May and the economic size (multiplier effect) of this figure exceeded TRY 600 Billion (HMB, 2020).

Especially credit packages were included in the development package. Loan packages have been created not only for businesses but also for individual uses. At this point, the Central Bank decided to reduce the policy interest by 100 basis points on March 18, 2020 in order to contribute to the healthy functioning of financial markets and to support the cash flow of the real sector. After this date, it reduced the policy interest rate to 8.25 % by making a total of 150 basis points reduction twice. Graph 8 contains interest rates since 2010.

In the COVID-19 process, in order to limit the negative effects of the pandemic on Turkey's economy, interest rates were cut to ensure that financial markets, credit channels and firms' cash flows continue to function in an uninterrupted and healthy manner. However, as a result of the rapid recovery achieved in the economy with strong credit momentum and developments in financial markets, inflation followed a higher course than expected. It was evaluated that the tightening steps taken since August should be strengthened in

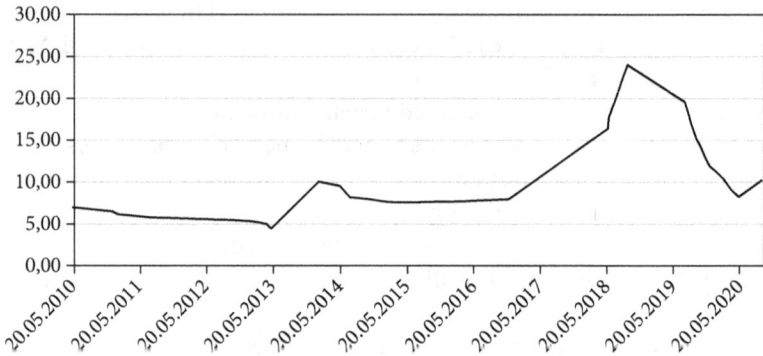

Graph 8. Policy interest rate (%). **Source:** It was created with data from the official website of the CBRT (CBRT, 2020 f)

order to control inflation expectations and limit the risks to the inflation out-look. Accordingly, the Monetary Policy Committee decided to raise the policy rate by 200 basis points on September 24, 2020 in order to restore the disinfla-tion process and support price stability (CBRT, 2020g). The steps of the CBRT essentially show that the problem is not one-sided. It has been shown that the necessary interventions should be made in a timely manner so that the steps taken to relieve the markets and give confidence to the investors are not more costly in the future. When the banking data published by the BRSA (2020) is considered, it is observed that there has been an increase of 27.2 % in total loans since the beginning of the year. This result may mean that the Central Bank's rate cut is equivalent in the real sector.

When the literature is examined, it is seen that lenders can support the company in cases of economic crisis and recession, if they have long-term relationships with companies and can access comprehensive information about them (Bolton et al., 2016, Beck et al., 2018). On the other hand, a longer slow-down or even a recession will put pressure on banks' loan portfolios and sol-vency positions. The reason for this pressure will be problem loans, a direct source of bank fragility. Unfortunately, such loan losses will not occur immedi-ately, they will not appear before late 2020 (Beck, 2020; 73–74).

Graph 9 gives statistics of non-performing loans as of January-July 2020. Until the pandemic process, a loan should have been 90 days late for a loan to be considered a non-performing loan. However, during this process, some banks offered their customers the opportunity to restructure their credits and

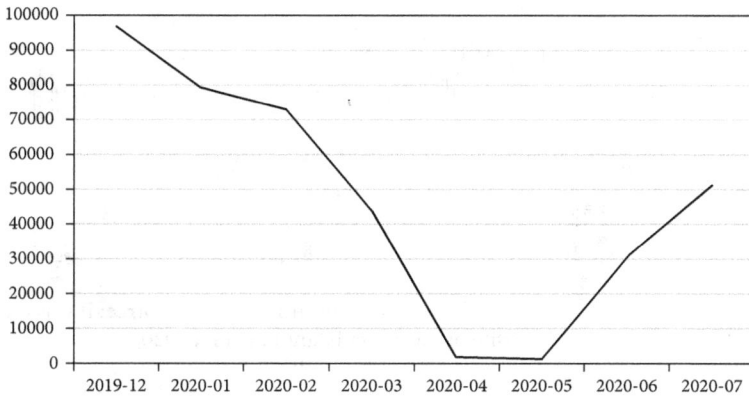

Graph 9. Non-performing loans (January-July 2020). **Source:** It was created with data from the official website of The Banks Association of Turkey (TBAT, 2020)

delay payments. Therefore, as seen in the Graph 9, new non-performing loans decreased considerably especially in April and May. In fact, delaying credit payments for an individual who is in financial trouble or unemployed may do nothing but delay the unhappy end. However, this opportunity provided to individuals and companies for the continuity of economic activities may be a reason for the effectiveness of financial markets.

Undoubtedly, non-performing loans are situations that banks never want to encounter. However, it is inevitable that loans will become problematic in the changing market environment and especially in times of extreme uncertainty such as the COVID-19 pandemic. Nkusu (2011) investigated the determinants of non-performing loans in the period 1998–2009. She found that worsening macroeconomic conditions, such as economic growth and high unemployment, led to higher non-performing loans. In this process, unemployment caused by companies that interrupt their production / services may cause an increase in non-performing loans. Banks may not be able to provide bridge financing for firms that have to cope with a sudden drop in demand. It may also decide that some businesses that are already in debt cannot cope with any additional short-term loans, which could result in businesses shutting down during the pandemic. For these reasons, it may be possible to see the reason behind the collapse of stock markets around the world. However, if many businesses are at financial risk due to the temporary decrease in social consumption, this primarily causes an increase in equity risk which helps explain the scope of the

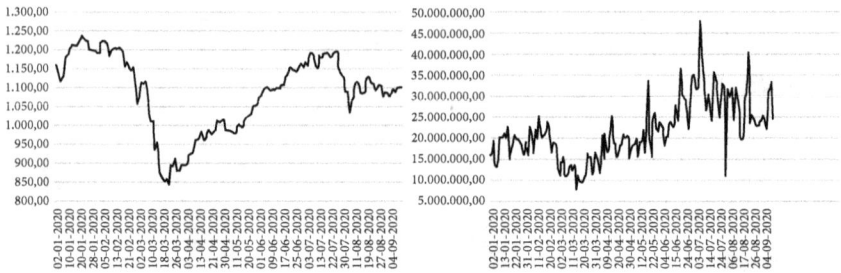

Graph 10. BIST 100 index and BIST 100 index trading volume. **Source:** It was created with data from the official website of the Borsa Istanbul (BIST, 2020)

stock market crash (Wren-Lewis, 2020; 111). To see the effect of the COVID-19 to stock market in Turkey is examined and BIST 100 Index and BIST 100 Index Trading Volume data.

Borsa İstanbul tested the levels of 1,100 and 1200 in January and February. COVID-19 first cases in Turkey are declared in the March 11, 2020. A day after the announcement, BIST suddenly fell from the levels of 1000s to the level of 936.40 with a decrease of 7.25 %. Although it is known that the markets are pricing expectations, the panic environment created by COVID-19 has caused investors to make rapid sales in an environment of uncertainty. The BIST 100 index, which experienced a decrease of about 10 % in the next week, started to rise again in line with the measures taken and the measures announced. In this process, it is thought that investors made quick sales in panic based on predictions, but they bought again due to the expectation of a quieter environment after the announcement of the measures. Similarly, China's Shanghai Composite, Hong Kong's Hang Seng, South Korea's KOSPI, Japan's Nikkei can be given as examples for the stock exchanges, which recovered in a short time after the announcement of support packages after a rapid fall. Similarly, Germany's DAX, England's FTSE 100 and Euro Stoxx 50 can all be cited as examples (Nicola, 2020).

2. Discussion

Although the measures taken to prevent the pandemic from spreading have an improving effect on public health, this pandemic also has an economic dimension. Namely, the process is inevitable that affect the not only Turkey but also entire world economy. As a result of the start and spread of the pandemic in China, the economic life in the country has come to a halt, as it is the second largest economy in the world, the economic changes in China affected almost the whole world in succession. Economy is not a univariate system. Therefore, In an economic system operating in a cycle, breaking of one link of the chain may cause the other rings to break.

Changes in macroeconomic indicators in the COVID-19 process are among the topics discussed in this study. With the fear of a new financial crisis and recession, many measures have been taken to relieve the market and restore economic balance. As the pandemic continues, new measures will continue to be taken. It is clearly seen here that the measures taken have a great impact not only on macroeconomic indicators but also on financial markets. In the COVID-19 process, in order to limit the negative effects of the pandemic on Turkey's economy, interest rates were cut to ensure that financial markets, credit channels and firms' cash flows continue to function in an uninterrupted and healthy manner. However, since financial troubles can not be improved with a single change, the rate cut, which relieved the markets for a while, prevented the disinflation process. For this reason, interest rates were raised again.

In this study, especially interrelated macroeconomic indicators are included and the rings that affect each other, including financial markets, are mentioned. In the crisis caused by COVID-19, taking steps that will have short-term consequences will provide temporary relief. The pandemic is still ongoing and the predictions for the end time are not very heartwarming. Therefore, financial institutions and the government need to constantly reassess the current situation. Medium and long-term planning are needed to revive the economy and achieve long-term prosperity. In fact, this process has shown that countries should also produce policies together. Therefore, common policies can be produced especially with countries with high trade volumes.

It is difficult to predict the impact of the COVID-19 crisis on the economy and financial markets in this uncertain environment. Therefore, in accordance with existing measures, the changes occurring in Turkey were explained on the basis of the data. Future studies can present the impact of the pandemic on macroeconomic indicators and financial markets with the help of time series.

References

Akiş, E. (2020), İktisadi Büyüme ve Kalkınma, İstanbul Üniversitesi Açık ve Uzaktan Eğitim Fakültesi İktisat Lisans Programı Ders Notu, http:// auzefkitap.istanbul.edu.tr/kitap/iktisat_ao/iktisadibuyumevekalk.pdf. Date of Access: 15.09.2020

Alisa, M. (2015), The Relationship between Inflation and Unemployment: A Theoretical Discussion about the Philips Curve, Journal of International Business and Economics, 3(2): 89–97.

Ay, S. (2012), Türkiye'de İşsizliğin Nedenleri: İstihdam Politikaları Üzerine Bir Değerlendirme, Yönetim ve Ekonomi, 19(2): 321–341.

Baldwin, R. and Mauro, W. (2020), Economics in the Time of COVID-19, A CEPR Press, London, UK.

Barışık, S. and Yayar, R. (2012), Sanayi Üretim Endeksini Etkileyen Faktörlerin Ekonometrik Analizi, İktisat İşletme ve Finans Dergisi, 27(316): 53–70.

Beck, T. (2020), Finance in the Times of Coronavirus, in Economics in the Time of COVID-19; ed. Richard Baldwin and Beatrice Weder di Mauro, CEPR Press, London, UK.

Beck, T., Degryse, H., Haas, R. D. and Horen, N. V. (2018), When Arm's Length Is too Far: Relationship Banking over the Credit Cycle, Journal of Financial Economics, 127(1): 174–196.

BIST (2020), Borsa Istanbul Equity Market Data, https://www.borsaistanbul.com/en/sayfa/3621/equity-market-data. Date of Access: 12.09.2020.

Bolton, P., Freixas, X., Gambacorta, L. and Mistrulli, P. E. (2016), Relationship and Transaction Lending in a Crisis, Review of Financial Studies, 29(10): 2643–2676.

BRSA (2020), Banking Regulation and Supervision Agency Monthly Banking Sector Data. https://www.bddk.org.tr/BultenAylik/en. Date of Access: 24.09.2020.

CBRT (2020a), Exchange Rates Datagroup, https://evds2.tcmb.gov.tr/index.php?/evds/serieMarket/#collapse_2. Date of Access: 17.09.2020.

CBRT (2020b), https://evds2.tcmb.gov.tr/index.php?/evds/serieMarket/collapse_18/5092/DataGroup/turkish/bie_ulusdovlkd/. Date of Access: 16.09.2020.

CBRT (2020c), https://tcmb.gov.tr/wps/wcm/connect/2b6d2e04-7e09-46cf-a14c-26683e436dc0/Foreign_Exchange_Reserve_Management2018.PDF?MOD=AJPERES. Date of Access: 15.09.2020.

CBRT (2020d), Company Accounts 2009–2019, http://www3.tcmb.gov.tr/sektor/2020/#/en. Date of Access: 17.09.2020.

CBRT (2020e), Survey of the Effects of the Pandemic on the Real Sector, https://www.tcmb.gov.tr/wps/wcm/connect/13002e0c-edb3-400a-b6b4-1e0aef372757/Box_4.2_2020_iii.pdf?MOD=AJPERES&CACHE=NONE&CONTENTCACHE=NONE. Date of Access: 16.09.2020.

CBRT (2020 f), Central Bank Interest Rates, https://www.tcmb.gov.tr/wps/wcm/connect/en/tcmb+en/main+menu/core+functions/monetary+policy/central+bank+interest+rates. Date of Access: 16.09.2020.

CBRT (2020g), Decision of the Monetary Policy Committee, https://tcmb.gov.tr/wps/wcm/connect/14c54ad8-ea7b-4509-9271-20685712da14/ANO2020-58.pdf?MOD=AJPERES&CACHEID=ROOTWORKSPACE-14c54ad8-ea7b-4509-9271-20685712da14-ni.NhXJ. Date of Access: 24.09.2020.

Eğilmez, M. (2020), Korona Virüsü ve İdlib Etkisi, Kendime Yazılar Blog, http://www.mahfiegilmez.com/2020/03/korona-virusu-ve-idlib-etkisi.html. Date of Access: 13.09.2020.

Grossman, G. M. and Krueger, A. B. (1995), Economic Growth and the Environment, The Quarterly Journal of Economics, 110(2): 353–377.

Güçlüoğlu, Ü. M. (2017), Türkiye İstihdam Analizi ve Bazı Makroekonomik Değişkenlerin İstihdam Üzerindeki Etkisi, Uzmanlık Tezi, Çalışma ve Sosyal Güvenlik Bakanlığı Türkiye İş Kurumu Genel Müdürlüğü, Ankara.

HMB (2020), T.C. Hazine ve Maliye Bakanlığı Basın Açıklaması, https://www.hmb.gov.tr/haberler/basin-aciklamasi. Date of Access: 13.09.2020.

IMF (2020a), World Economic Outlook the Great Lockdown, April-2020, https://www.imf.org/en/Publications/WEO/Issues/2020/04/14/World-Economic-Outlook-April-2020-The-Great-Lockdown-49306. Date of Access: 14.09.2020.

IMF (2020b), A Crisis Like No Other, An Uncertain Recovery, World Economic Outlook Update-June 2020, https://www.imf.org/en/Publications/WEO/Issues/2020/06/24/WEOUpdateJune2020. Date of Access: 16.09.2020.

Jones, C. I., Spence Takes, M. and Spence, M. (1998), Introduction of Economic Growth, W.W. Norton & Co, New York.

Li, X., Meng, B. Wang, Z. (2019), Recent Patterns of Global Production and GVC Participation, in Technological Innovation, Supply Chain Trade, and Workers in a Globalized World- Global Value Chain Development Report 2019, 9-44, Switzerland.

McKibbin, W. J. and Fernando, R. (2020), The Global Macroeconomic Impacts of COVID-19: Seven Scenarios, CAMA Working Paper No. 19/2020.

MoC (2020), Covid-19 Gelişmeleri, https://ticaret.gov.tr/yurtdisi-teskilati/dogu-asya/cin-halk-cumhuriyeti/ulke-profili/covid-19-gelismeleri. Date of Access: 14.09.2020.

MoH (2020), General Coronavirus Table, https://covid19.saglik.gov.tr/TR-66935/genel-koronavirus-tablosu.html. Date of Access: 11.09.2020.

Nicola, M., Alsafi, Z., Sohrabi, C., Kerwan, A., Al-Jabir, A., Iosifidis, C., Agha, M. and Agha, R. (2020), The Socio-Economic Implications of the Coronavirus Pandemic (COVID-19): A Review, Elsevier Public Health Emergency Collection, 78: 185–193.

Nkusu, M. (2011), Nonperforming Loans and Macrofinancial Vulnerabilities in Advanced Economies, IMF Working Paper, WP/11/161: 1–27.

Onaran, Ö. (2002), Measuring Wage Flexibility: The Case of Turkey before and after Structural Adjustment, Applied Economics, 34(6): 767–781.

Oskooe, S. A. P. (2010), Emerging Stock Market Performance and Economic Growth, American Journal of Applied Sciences, 7(2): 265–269.

Pal, R. (2018), Economic Growth, Inflation and Unemployment, in Issues and Concepts of Economics, Adhyayan Publishers and Distributors, New Delhi.

Phillips, A.W. (1958), The Relationship between Unemployment and the Rate of Change of Money Wage Rates in the United Kingdom, 1861–1957, Economica, New Series, 25(100): 283–299.

PIO (2020), News from Turkey, Presidency of the Republic of Turkey Investment Office, https://www.invest.gov.tr/en/news/news-from-turkey/pages/president-erdogan-unveils-economic-stability-shield-program.aspx. Date of Access: 14.09.2020.

Qun Li, M., Guan, X., Wu, P. et al. (2020), Early Transmission Dynamics in Wuhan, China, of Novel Coronavirus–Infected Pneumonia, The New England Journal of Medicine, 382(13): 1199–1207.

Resmi Gazete (2003), 4857 Sayılı İş Kanunu, https://www.mevzuat.gov.tr/MevzuatMetin/1.5.4857.pdf. Date of Access: 16.09.2020.

Resmi Gazete (2011), 6111 Sayılı Bazı Alacakların Yeniden Yapılandırılması ile Sosyal Sigortalar ve Genel Sağlık Sigortası Kanunu ve Diğer Bazı Kanun ve Kanun Hükmünde Kararnamelerde Değişiklik Yapılması Hakkında Kanun, https://www.resmigazete.gov.tr/eskiler/2011/02/20110225M1-1.htm. Date of Access: 16.09.2020.

Resmi Gazete (2020), 7244 SayılıYeni Koronavirüs (COVID-19) Salgınının Ekonomik ve Sosyal Hayata Etkilerinin Azaltılması Hakkında Kanun ile Bazı Kanunlarda Değişiklik Yapılmasına Dair Kanun, https://www.resmigazete.gov.tr/eskiler/2020/04/20200417-2.htm. Date of Access: 16.09.2020.

TBAT (2020), The Banks Association of Turkey, https://verisistemi.tbb.org.tr/index.php?/tbb/report_rm. Date of Access: 16.09.2020.

Terzi, H. and Oltulular, S. (2004), Türkiye'de Sanayileşme ve Ekonomik Büyüme Arasındaki Nedensel İlişki, Doğuş Üniversitesi Dergisi, 5(2): 219–226.

Turkstat (2020a), Turkish Statistical Institute Foreign Trade Indices, July 2020, http://www.turkstat.gov.tr/PreHaberBultenleri.do?id=33843. Date of Access: 15.09.2020.

Turkstat (2020b), Turkish Statistical Institute Foreign Trade Statistics, July 2020, http://www.turkstat.gov.tr/PreHaberBultenleri.do?id=33855. Date of Access: 15.09.2020.

Turkstat (2020c), Turkish Statistical Institute Industrial Production Index, July 2020, http://www.turkstat.gov.tr/HbGetirHTML.do?id=33802. Date of Access: 15.09.2020.

Turkstat (2020d), Turkish Statistical Institute Quarterly Gross Domestic Product, Quarter II: April-June, 2020, http://www.turkstat.gov.tr/ HbGetirHTML.do?id=33605. Date of Access: 16.09.2020.

Turkstat (2020e), Turkish Statistical Institute Labour Force Statistics, June 2020, http://www.turkstat.gov.tr/HbGetirHTML.do?id=33790. Date of Access: 16.09.2020.

Turkstat (2020 f), Turkish Statistical Institute Consumer Price Index, August 2020, http://www.turkstat.gov.tr/HbGetirHTML.do?id=33869. Date of Access: 16.09.2020.

Türkiş (2020), Ağustos 2020 Açlık ve Yoksulluk Sınırı, http://www.turkis.org. tr/AGUSTOS-2020-ACLIK-VE-YOKSULLUK-SINIRI-d435750. Date of Access: 16.09.2020.

WHO (2020), Archived: WHO Timeline – COVID-19, https://www.who. int/news-room/detail/27-04-2020-who-timeline---covid-19. Date of Access: 05.09.2020.

Wren-Lewis, S. (2020), The Economic Effects of a Pandemic, in Economics in the Time of COVID-19; ed. Richard Baldwin and Beatrice Weder di Mauro, CEPR Press, London, UK.

Yorulmaz, R. and Kaptan, S. (2020), Kovid-19 ile Mücadele Sürecinde Maliye Politikalarının Rolü, in Kovid-19 (Koronavirüs) Salgınının Ekonomik Etkileri, ed. İbrahim Demir, Ulisa12, Ankara.

Asst. Prof. Hüseyin Başar Önem

Business Capital Elements before and after COVID-19 Pandemic: A Study on Borsa İstanbul Pharmaceutical-Health Shares

1. Introduction

Coronaviruses (CoV) are a large family of viruses that cause a variety of illnesses, from the common cold to more serious diseases such as Middle East Respiratory Syndrome (MERS-CoV) and Severe Acute Respiratory Syndrome (SARS-CoV). The WHO China Country Office reported cases of pneumonia of unknown etiology in Wuhan, China's Hubei province, on December 31, 2019. On January 7, 2020, the agent was identified as a new coronavirus (2019-nCoV) that was not previously detected in humans (Turkish Ministry of Health, 2020).

This virus, which has a very high rate of transmission, appeared in Turkey with the first case on March 11, 2020 (Budak & Korkmaz, 2020). To minimize economic destruction due to the COVID-19 pandemic, some regulations were made in Turkey and various support packages were announced (Keleş, 2020). Furthermore, curfews and the closure of some workplaces at certain times or completely have been a continuation of the measures. Increasing these precautions have also caused fluctuations in businesses economically.

According to the Central Bank of the Republic of Turkey, while the COVID-19 pandemic has caused a serious health threat on the global world scale, it has also had a major impact on the countries' economies. Precautions to prevent the spread of the COVID-19 pandemic negatively affect people's consumption habits, manufacturing processes, and employment of enterprises (Central Bank of the Republic of Turkey, 2020). With this virus spreading around the world, many problems have arisen in economic, social, etc. These problems have caused great economic difficulties on a micro and macro scale. The COVID-19 pandemic, which has been affected all over the world, has been observed to have greater economic effects than the financial crisis on a global scale in 2008 (Adıgüzel, 2020). To control the effects of the pandemic in all countries, governments have uncovered various practices. On the one hand, central banks are attempting to provide liquidity to countries, while on the other hand precautions are being taken to support several households and businesses with high financial policies and the effects of the pandemic (Central Bank of the Republic of Turkey, 2020).

It is thought that the change and transformation of countries due to their economic, financial, and commercial structures will continue in the processes after the pandemic. The change and transformation caused by the pandemic holds risks and threats all over the world, as well as alternatives and opportunities, according to the structure of each country (Korkut, 2020).

Assets used to sustain the business operations and reaching liquidity in a short time are defined as working capital (Çakır & Küçükkaplan, 2012). The concept of business capital management is also called working capital management. Working capital management includes the number of assets available, the financing of these assets, and the decision of this composition (Dalayeen, 2017). The financing of the business capital, which is cashed out in a short time, can be made from different balance sheet items. In other words, the concept of working capital management includes decisions about financing a certain amount of the business's investment in rotating assets with short-term external resources and how much of the returned assets will be financed with long-term external resources and equity (Akel & İltaş, 2016). The concept of business capital management is directly related to the liquidity and profitability of firms (Raheman & Nasr, 2007). The purpose of business capital management is to ensure the optimum balance of each of the components of business capital (Filbeck & Krueger, 2006). Due to the increase in the costs of operations under current conditions, the management of business capital has become more important for the survival of a company. Key elements of business capital are current assets and current debts (Iqbal & Zhuquan, 2015). Business capital management plays an important role in success or failure in the business world due to its impact on firm profitability and liquidity (Dong & Su, 2010). Firstly, the company's profits do not fall with effective business capital management. Secondly, the speed of cash circulation increases, and ultimately costs fall (Alipour, 2011).

Outbreaks occurring around the world or in countries are also a kind of crisis. Businesses are often severely affected by working capital management crisis environments. Deterioration of the cash structure, changes in receivables and inventory amounts, difficulties in debt payment power, and other liquidity declines are some of the problems seen as business capital management in a crisis environment.

The aim of this study is to reveal by years the changes of business capital elements of companies in Borsa Istanbul Pharmaceutical-Health sector before and after the COVID-19 pandemic period. It will also contribute to the literature if the COVID-19 pandemic process continues, or in new outbreaks, business managers are prepared for this financial situation.

2. Methods

In this study, business capital elements before and after the COVID-19 pandemic period were examined. In this context, 5 companies in Borsa Istanbul Pharmaceutical-Health sector were included in the study. Related companies are DEVA Holding A.Ş., EİS Eczacıbaşı İlaç, Sınai ve Finansal Yatırımlar Sanayi ve Ticaret A.Ş., Lokman Hekim Engürüsağ Sağlık Turizm Eğitim Hizmetleri ve İnşaat Taahhüt A.Ş., RTA Laboratuvarları Biyolojik Ürünler İlaç ve Makine Sanayi Ticaret A.Ş., and Selçuk Ecza Deposu Ticaret ve Sanayi A.Ş. Pharmaceutical-Health sector companies traded on Borsa İstanbul in the years before 2015 were based on data from 2015 and later because there were not enough and their information could not be accessed. It was calculated the effects of the COVID-19 pandemic on the business capital of these companies by taking the average of the current ratio, acid-test ratio, cash ratio, and liquidity ratios between the first and second quarters of 2015–2020 (Eljelly, 2004; Christopher & Kamalavalli, 2009; Kendirli & Konak, 2014) with the receivable turnover ratio and the stock turnover ratio from the operating ratios (Çakır & Küçükkaplan, 2012). All data used in the study were obtained from public financial tables in PDP (Public Disclosure Platform) website.

Three ratios for liquidity ratios and two rates for activity rates were used in the study. The current rate is calculated by dividing the total current assets of enterprises into short-term external resources. It shows the firm's ability to pay short-term debts. The acid-test rate, the liquid ratio in other words, is calculated by taking out stocks from current assets and dividing them into short-term debts to more accurately calculate whether businesses can pay their short-term debts compared to the current rate. The cash rate is the most reliable liquidity rate that reveals the financial situation of the firm. It is calculated by dividing the sum of liquid assets and securities into current assets. Besides, stock turnover rate and receivables turnover ratios from operating rates, which are extremely important as business capital management, are included in the calculation. The proportions that show the extent to which businesses' assets are used efficiently are operating rates. The stock turnover rate is the rate at which businesses' stocks are renewed and sold several times in a year. The stock turnover rate is the rate at how many times businesses' stocks are renewed and sold in a year. The stock turnover rate is calculated by dividing the cost of the sold goods by the average inventory quantity. The rate of receivables turnover is the rate at which receivables are collected several times in a year, and it is calculated by dividing credit sales into average trade receivables.

3. Results

According to Fig. 1, when the data for the current rate in the first quarters are examined, the highest rate is the first quarter of 2018 and the lowest current rate is the first quarter of 2020. Looking at the data in the second quarters, it is also seen that the highest year is 2018 and the lowest current rate is in 2017. In 2018–2020 years, there was a sharp fall.

Overall, looking at the results of the first quarter and second quarter, the results are close together, but in 2019, the first quarter current rate is more de-separated than the second quarter. According to the results of the first quarter and second quarter of 2020, which is the COVID-19 pandemic period, there is a drop in the current rate.

According to Fig. 2, the acid-test ratio in the first quarter is the highest in 2018 and the lowest is 2016. When looking at the data in the second quarters, it is also seen that the highest year is 2018 and the lowest acid-test ratio is in 2017. Looking in general, the biggest decomposition was in 2019, as was the current rate. According to the results of the first-quarter and the second-quarter of 2020, which is the pandemic period, there was a drop in the acid-test ratio.

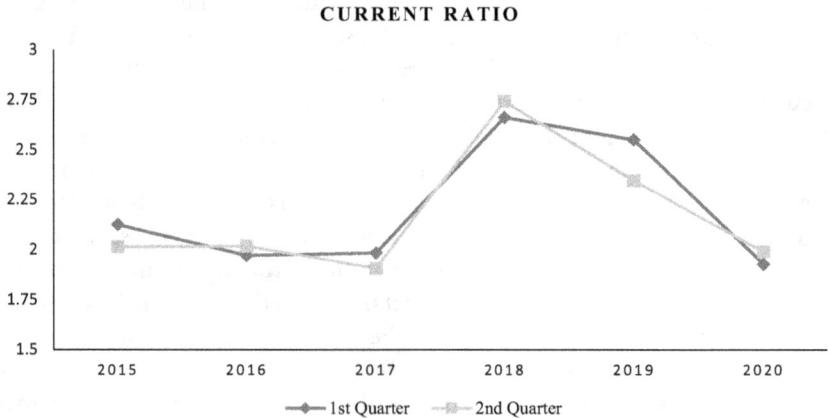

Fig. 1. Findings on current ratios of enterprises

ACID TEST RATIO

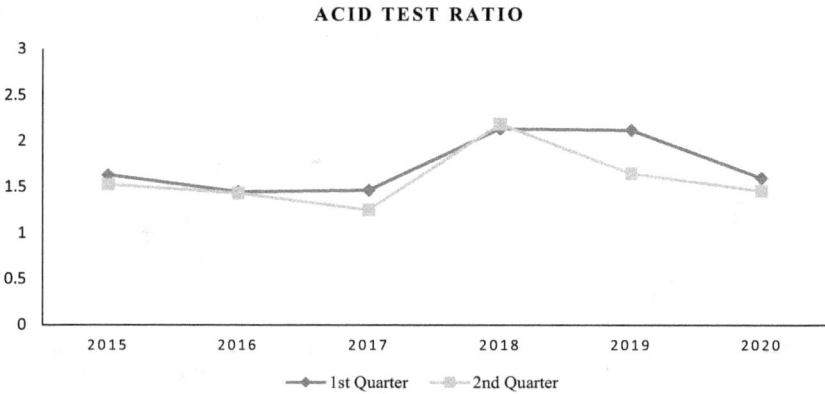

Fig. 2. Findings on acid-test ratios of enterprises

CASH RATE

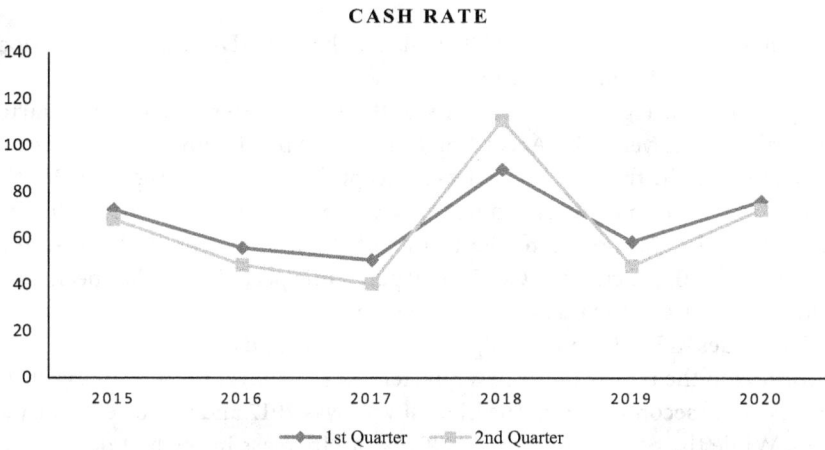

Fig. 3. Findings on cash rates of enterprises

According to Fig. 3, when the data for the cash rate in the first quarters are examined, the highest year is 2018 and the lowest year is 2017. Looking at the results of the second quarter, the highest year is 2018 and the lowest year is 2017. Looking in general, the results of the first-quarter cash rate are lower than the second-quarter results except for 2018. According to the results of the first

RECEIVABLES TURNOVER

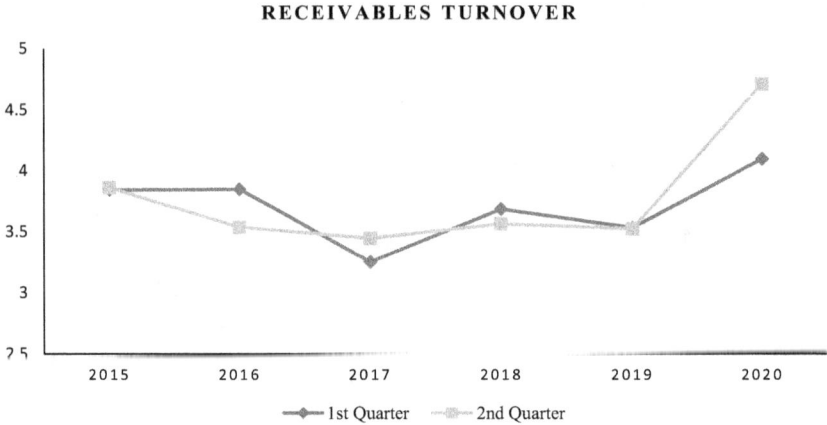

Fig. 4. Findings on receivables turnover ratios of enterprises

quarter and second quarter of 2020, which is the COVID-19 pandemic period, there was a drop in the cash ratio.

The values in Fig. 4 are the results of the first quarter and second quarter receivables turnover ratio. According to these results, in 2015–2020, there are similar values in the rate of turnover except for 2020. Looking at 2020, the results of the second quarter have increased significantly compared to first quarter results. According to the results of the first quarter and the second quarter of 2020, which is the COVID-19 pandemic period, there has been a significant increase in the rate of receivables turnover.

The values in Fig. 5 were the highest year in 2017 and the lowest year in 2020, according to the results of the first quarter stock turnover ratio. Looking at the results of the second quarter, the highest year was 2017 and the lowest year was 2019. While the pandemic period 2020 was an increase in the first quarter, according to the results of the second quarter there was a significant drop in the stock turnover ratio.

4. Discussion

In this study, the values of business capital elements that have a very important place for business finance during the COVID-19 pandemic period were compared to the years before the COVID-19 pandemic. There were no studies on business capital management and published during the COVID-19 pandemic in the literature. In this regard, it is thought that the study will contribute to the

STOCK TURNOVER

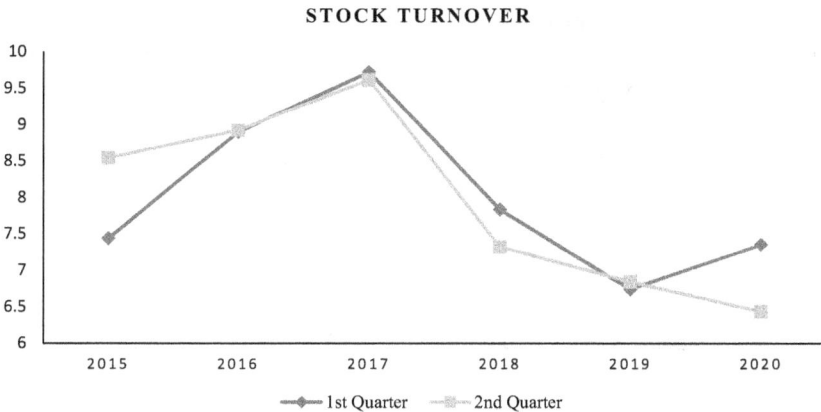

Fig. 5. Findings on stock turnover ratios of enterprises

literature. However, many studies have been carried out before the pandemic period related to business capital management. In this chapter, evaluations of business capital elements were made during and before the COVID-19 pandemic. The inclusion of sampling of five companies related to the COVID-19 pandemic period traded on the Borsa Istanbul and the utilization of first-quarter and second-quarter data in 2015–2020 years should be considered as a significant constraint of the study.

According to the findings of the study, the current rate and acid-test ratio decreased during the COVID-19 pandemic period compared to the previous two years. This may mean that businesses involved in the analysis may have trouble paying short-term external resources with their current assets if the COVID-19 pandemic continues. When looking at the cash rate, there has been an increase compared to the year before the COVID-19 pandemic. The 2018 year at the cash rate was the highest. Turkey's economy grew 7.2 % in the first quarter of the year and 5.3 % in the second quarter in 2018 are likely to occur as a result of such a rate (T.R. Presidency of the Strategy and Budget, 2018). The results of the COVID-19 pandemic period have reached their highest level according to other years in the rate of receivables turnover. The high rate of receivables turnover causes the collection capacity of the enterprises is positive, thus businesses to be more comfortable repaying debts during the COVID-19 pandemic (Akgün, 2002). The first quarter of the COVID-19 pandemic period is higher than the second quarter in terms of the stock turnover rate. At the same time, the COVID-19 pandemic period between first and second-quarter data is lower in terms of stock turnover rate than other years. Falling stock turnover is not a pleasant situation, and this may mean that the business is having trouble cashing in its stocks.

As a result, this study fills a significant gap in the literature by demonstrating how the business capital management elements of enterprises act in pandemic periods. It is thought that this study will be an important indicator for business managers in the event of a continued pandemic or future outbreaks.

References

Adıgüzel, M. (2020). COVID-19 Pandemisinin Türkiye ekonomisine etkilerinin makroekonomik analizi. İstanbul Ticaret Üniversitesi Sosyal Bilimler Dergisi Covid-19 Sosyal Bilimler Özel Sayısı, Bahar (Özel Ek), 191–221.

Akgün, M. (2002). İşletmelerde etkinlik ve nakit çevirme süresi analizi, Mali Çözüm, Sayı:60, Yıl:12.

Alipour, M. (2011). Working capital management and corporate profitability: Evidence from Iran, World Applied Sciences Journal, 12 (7), 1093–1099.

Budak, F. & Korkmaz, Ş. (2020). COVID-19 pandemi sürecine yönelik genel bir değerlendirme: Türkiye örneği. Sosyal Araştırmalar ve Yönetim Dergisi, (1), 62–79.

Central Bank of the Republic of Turkey. (2020). Koronavirüsün ekonomik ve finansal etkilerine karşı alınan tedbirler, koronavirüs ve ekonomi. https://www.tcmb.gov.tr/wps/wcm/connect/TR/TCMB+TR/Main+Menu/Duyurular/Koronavirus.

Christopher, S. B. & Kamalavalli, A. L. (2009), Sensitivity of profitability to working capital management in Indian corporate hospitals, International Journal of Managerial and Financial Accounting, 213–227.

Çakır, H. M. & Küçükkaplan, İ. (2012). İşletme sermayesi unsurlarının firma değeri ve karlılığı üzerindeki etkisinin İMKB'de işlem gören üretim firmalarında 2000 – 2009 dönemi için analiz. Muhasebe ve Finansman Dergisi, 69–86.

Dalayeen, B. A. (2017). Working capital management and profitability of real estate industry in Jordan: An empirical study, Journal of Applied Finance & Banking, 7(2), 49–57.

Dong, H. P. & Su, J. (2010). The relationship between working capital management and profitability: A Vietnam case, International Research Journal of Finance and Economics, (49), 59–67.

Eljelly, A. (2004). Liquidity-profitability tradeoff: An empirical investigation in an emerging market, International Journal of Commerce & Management, 14(2), 48–61. https://doi.org/10.1108/10569210480000179

Filbeck, G. & Krueger, T. M. (2006). An analysis of working capital management results across industries, Mid-American Journal of Business, 20(2), 11–18. https://doi.org/10.1108/19355181200500007

Iqbal, A. & Zhuquan, W. (2015). Working capital management and profitability evidence from firms listed on Karachi stock Exchange, International Journal of Business and Management, 10(2), 231–235. doi:10.5539/ijbm.v10n2p231

Keleş, E. (2020). COVID-19 ve BİST-30 Endeksi üzerine kısa dönemli etkileri. Marmara Üniversitesi İktisadi ve İdari Bilimler Dergisi, 91–105.

Korkut, C. (2020). Küresel salgın sonrasında ekonomi ve finansta Türkiye: alternatifler ve fırsatlar, küresel salgının anatomisi: İnsan ve toplumun geleceği, Türkiye Bilimler Akademisi, 563–584.

Raheman, A. & Nasr, M. (2007). Working capital management and profitability case of Pakistani firms, International Review of Business Research Papers, 3(1), 279–300.

Turkish Ministry of Health, Halk Sağlığı Genel Müdürlüğü. (2020). 2019-nCoV hastalığı sağlık çalışanları rehberi. Bilim Kurulu Çalışması. https://hsgm. saglik.gov.tr/depo/haberler/ncov/2019-nCov_Hastal_Salk_alanlar_Rehberi. pdf, Access date: 25.09.2020.

T.R. Presidency of the Strategy and Budget. (2018). Ekonomik Gelişmeler (2018 yılı 3. çeyrek), Aralık-2018. http://www.sbb.gov.tr/wp-content/ uploads/2018/12/2018-Ekonomik-Geli%C5 %9Fmeler-3-Ceyrek.pdf, Access date: 23.09.2020.

Asst. Prof. Serap Taşkaya

COVID-19 Pandemic and Healthcare Workforce: A Bibliometric Study

1. Introduction

Coronaviruses are the types of viruses that can cause serious lower respiratory tract infections such as pneumonia and bronchiolitis, as well as upper respiratory tract infections. Two types of infections in humans were first described in the 1960s. In 2003, a new type of coronavirus was found in "Severe Acute Respiratory Syndrome" (SARS) cases that caused a pandemic for the first time. In 2004 and 2005, two new types of coronavirus were also found that commonly cause respiratory infections in humans. In 2012, the world met the novel coronavirus called "Middle East Respiratory Syndrome" (MERS). Unlike SARS and MERS, the coronavirus types encountered in 1960 and 2004–2005 generally caused mild to moderate infections (Nemli and Demirdal, 2016: 78).

COVID-19 is the newest coronavirus infection, which can be associated with occasional dry cough, weakness, difficulty breathing and vomiting etc. (Zhou et al., 2020: 1). After its first appearance in December 2019 in China, a series of articles detailing the disease were published within a few weeks trying to define the epidemiology of the disease. The virus was identified and typed in early January 2020. This type of virus shares 79 % identity with the SARS coronavirus and 50 % with the MERS coronavirus (Park et al., 2020: 308). However, it was soon realized that this novel coronavirus was very different from SARS and MERS. For example, while both older types of coronavirus are associated primarily with nosocomial and a low risk of transmission, COVID-19 appears to be much more common in the community and is transmitted by human to human contact (Petrosillo, 2020: 730).

Compared with SARS and MERS, COVID-19 has spread more quickly in the world, partially due to increased globalization and epidemiological emphasis but has lower fatality (Singhal, 2020: 281). At the end of the SARS outbreak, more than 8,000 cases of illness and 774 deaths were recorded with a fatality rate of 7 %. Since 2012, the reported MERS cases are 2494, and the associated deaths are 858 with a 34.4 % case-fatality ratio (Peeri et al., 2020: 2–7). On the other hand, the World Health Organization reported nearly 22 million confirmed cases and 800.000 deaths with a 1 % case-fatality ratio at the end of

August 2020 (World Health Organization, 2020a: 1). Many of the cases are still either quarantined or isolated (Itodo et al., 2020: 534).

In addition to health problems such as death and illness, COVID-19 has affected almost all aspects of daily life, causing involuntary alienation and separation, economic difficulties, fear of a life-threatening illness and feelings of helplessness (Polizzi et al., 2020: 59). With no effective vaccination or cure available, most policymakers have implemented lockdowns to curb the virus' development. These aggressive health policies a decrease in domestic production and a decrease in national income. In the global sense, it is thought that the world will experience a global economic crisis, high inflation and high unemployment rates due to the lack of production during and after the pandemic. In this context, in order to face less harm after the pandemic, every country should take measures to balance the health demand and the needs of its people, regardless of the socio-economic situation (Buheji et al., 2020: 213).

As mentioned above, the COVID-19 epidemic triggered an ongoing social and economic crisis, especially in the service sectors (Bartsch et al., 2020: 1). Today, services constitute a large part of economic outputs, foreign investments and world trade. Social distance and mobility restriction applied during the pandemic period affected the services based on physical proximity between the producer and the consumer the most. For example, sectors such as retail services, tourism and passenger transportation stopped their production in this period. The decrease in the production of services in these sectors has made decisions regarding both the existing transactions in the domestic and foreign markets and the establishment of new institutions negative. Therefore, from the perspective of a country's economy, it is evident that disruptions in the supply of services will cause significant reductions in trade and other economic activities, and inequalities in social and economic inclusion (World Trade Organization, 2020: 1). Finally, organizations that provide vital infrastructures such as healthcare, distribution and food retailing have started to take appropriate protective measures to protect consumers and especially their employees (Bartsch et al., 2020: 2).

The COVID-19 pandemic has affected the entire service industry, but the health sector, as the epicenter of the virus has been most seriously impacted around worldwide. In many nations, health services are being overreached with growing cases (Etyang, 2020: 1). When the number of people affected by COVID-19 rises, the healthcare system has been overburdened. Besides COVID-19 patients, there are other patients they still have to care for, such as diabetes, blood pressure, cancer, liver and kidney failure (Zaki et al., 2020: 1134). As a result, serious resource constraints have been encountered such lack of personal protection devices, insufficient intensive care beds and personnel shortage to care for seriously ill patients (Hoffmann et al., 2020: 179). Of these inadequate resources, the most important is the health workforce, which is considered the central part and heart of every health system (International Labour Organisation, 2020a: 1).

The unexpected and accelerated dissemination of the COVID-19 pandemic around the world has triggered a drastic change in the work environment of health care staff (Bostan et al., 2020: 1). Health workers have always been the group with the highest risk of being caught against pandemic factors (Tuncay et al., 2020: 489). Especially doctors and nurses in the affected countries are serving at high risk of infection and under hard working conditions (Wu et al., 2020: 60). In addition to the insufficient personal protective equipment, the lack of awareness of the healthcare professionals on protection devices, the long-term exposure to many infected patients, and the lack of education about the pandemic increased the risk of infection for healthcare workers (Wang et al., 2020: 1). As a result, even at the end of May, which is considered to be the early stages of the disease, it had been reported that more than one hundred and fifty thousand healthcare personnel were infected, and approximately one thousand five hundred of them died (Bandyopadhyay et al., 2020: 8). Infection of healthcare professionals while working at work is also a significant problem, as it may cause the virus to be transmitted to colleagues, families, friends, and others (International Labour Organisation, 2020b: 6).

In addition to increasing mortality and morbidity rates, during the COVID-19 epidemic, healthcare staff became significantly at risk for adverse effects in physical and mental well-being. Digestive disturbances, weight changes, allergic responses, fatigue, vomiting, muscle and heart problems are among the concerns with physical health. Poor mood, low energy, exhaustion, anxiety, stress, burnout, irritability, suicidal behavior, and elevated substance use, such as cigarettes, alcohol, and medications, are examples of mental disorders (International Labour Organisation, 2020b: 6). Long hours of work, risk of illness, insufficient medical supplies, loneliness, tiredness and family break are all reasons for that issues (Kang et at., 2020: 14; Rajkumar, 2020: 3). Also, increased stress, emotional fatigue, nosocomial delivery and the need to make complicated choices on treatment issues may have drastic consequences on their physical and mental health (Pappa et al., 2020: 901). These health issues not only hinder caregiver focus, understanding, decision-making and the fight against COVID-19 but can also have a significant influence on overall well-being. Therefore, improving the health of healthcare professionals during the pandemic period helps prevent diseases and achieve sustainable health goals (Kang et at., 2020: 14).

COVID-19 also has a direct effect on the workplace atmosphere of health-care professionals and causes changes in their organizational behavior (International Labour Organisation, 2020b: 7). Organizational factors such as the sudden increase in workload, long hours of work, and low rest periods, and the personal characteristics of healthcare professionals such as age, gender, race, ethnic origin and culture differentiate their attitudes towards their organizations (Kniffin et al., 2020: 5). Work-related concerns also include the existence of unclear rules, inadequate information delivery, and lack of feedback channels in pandemic periods (Fu et al., 2020: 3193). All these factors change the organizational perceptions of health professionals like leadership, communication, safety, climate and support, etc. (Burton, 2010: 26) and ultimately leads to an increase in absenteeism, presenteeism and turnover intention and a decrease in employee satisfaction, commitment, and productivity (International Labour Organisation, 2020b: 14).

Health professionals perform a vital role not only in the diagnosis and treatment of patients but also in ensuring that effective preventive and safety strategies are applied in health care facilities. Therefore, understanding the relationship between COVID-19 infection and healthcare professionals is the most accurate step in reducing the spread of the disease and preventing future infections (World Health Organization, 2020b: 5). However, when the studies conducted are examined, it is noticed that the general evaluations regarding the COVID-19 pandemic and healthcare staff in the current literature are almost negligible (Labrague and De los Santos, 2020: 2–3; Spoorthy et al., 2020: 1). Hence, this study was conducted to assess associations between COVID-19 and healthcare workforce. The research plans to provide an overview of studies investigating this issue using a bibliometric method. The results obtained from the research are expected to give an idea of which studies have been done more in this field and which studies have been less.

2. Methods

The bibliometric method, which examines certain elements of academic articles through statistical and numerical analysis, was first introduced to the literature in 1969 by Alan Pritchard. It is concerned with the statistical analysis of data of scientific research and studies such as discipline, subject, author, publication information, citation information, institution and country. The results obtained with this method give a general perspective of a particular discipline (Okubo, 1997: 8–9). In this study, the presentation of a broad summary of the studies examining the effect of COVID-19 on healthcare workers was carried out with bibliometric analysis.

In every bibliometric analysis, the first step is to determine which archive is suitable to use to collect the necessary records (Sweileh, 2020: 3). Today, there are many databases such as Web of Science, Scopus, Google Scholar, PubMed, MEDLINE can be used for bibliometric research to obtain data. However, Web of Science is frequently used in the bibliometric analysis because it covers many journals and provides excellent convenience for researchers (Demir and Erigüç, 2018: 95; Wei, 2019: 27). So Web of Science was used to fulfill the research goal in the present study.

The second step in a bibliometric study is to create a valid search query that will take as many documents as possible and have the least irrelevant results (Sweileh, 2020: 3). In this study, a detailed literature search had been made for the selection of the query words and the following search terms were used: (COVID-19 OR SARS-COV-2 OR coronavirus) AND (healthcare employee* OR health care employee* OR medical employee* OR health care worker* OR healthcare worker* OR medical worker* OR health care specialist* healthcare specialist* OR medical specialist*OR healthcare professional* OR medical professional* OR health care professional* OR health care professions* OR professions* OR medical professions* OR health care workforce* OR healthcare workforce* OR medical workforce* OR health care staff* healthcare staff* medical staff* hospital staff* OR physician* OR doctor* OR general practitioner* OR nurse* OR midwife* OR dentist* OR pharmacist* OR healthcare manager* Or health care manager* OR healthcare provider* OR health care provider*).

The above-mentioned query words were scanned in the title area of all studies without any restrictions in the WoS database. The most used approach in the validation of search queries is based on making the same query by another author and comparing the obtained articles. The comparison is made using the Pearson correlation test. A significant and strong correlation is indicative of the high validity of the search query (Sweileh, 2020: 3). For this research, another researcher conducted a literature search using the same query words and the reliability of both queries were found as 0.96. In short, it can be said that the data used for the study were reliable.

The Web of Science search for this study was carried out on 09.09.2020. The search query found out 37.997 documents on COVID-19 literature and 820 of them about human resources for health. The titles, keywords and abstracts of all publications had been examined and 22 publications were removed because they were related to MERS or SARS. Also, 69 of them were excluded because they were news items (n=68) and reprinted (N=1). Finally, the analysis was

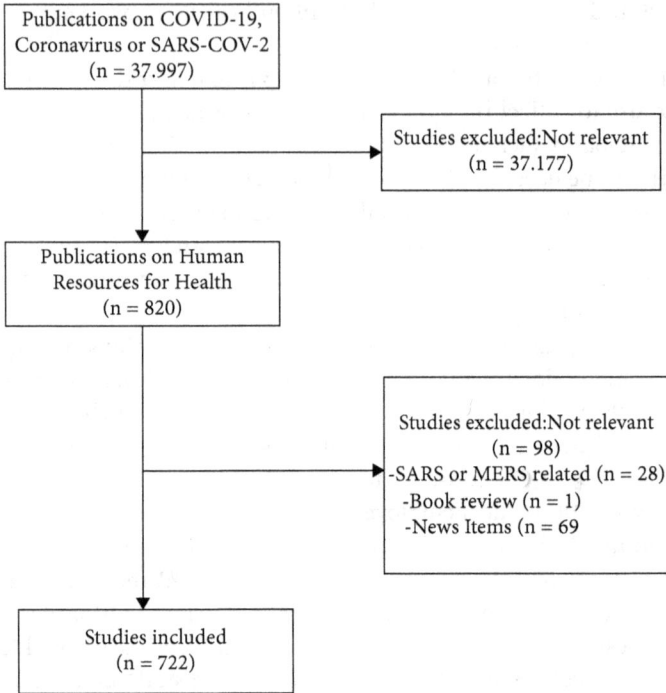

Fig. 1. Information on the selection of publications used in the study

ultimately carried out on 722 documents. Information on all these stages can be found in Fig. 1.

In this study, publications on the effects of COVID-19 on healthcare workers were classified and evaluated according to the parameters "document type," "language," "country of origin," "organization," " subject area,"" source title," "citation," and "co-word." The tables in the result part were created using the Microsoft Excel program. For figures, the VOS viewer, which helps to create and visualize bibliometric networks, was used and each document was loaded into this program.

3. Results

This study, which is on the relationship between COVID-19 and human resources for health, is based on a total of 722 publications. Fig. 2 contains information on the types of publications. Accordingly, 42 % of all publications are

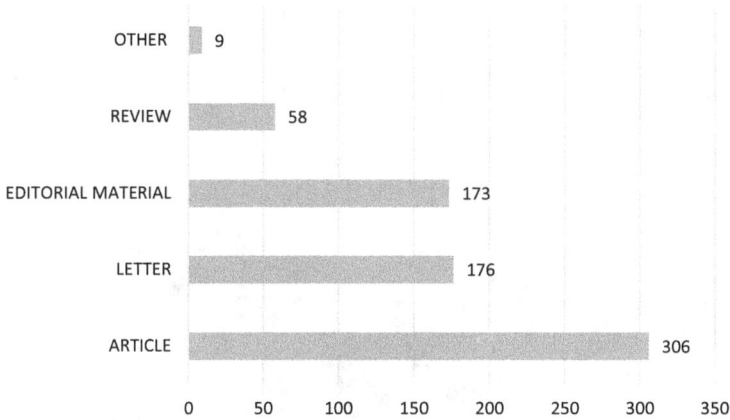

Fig. 2. Distribution of the types of publications

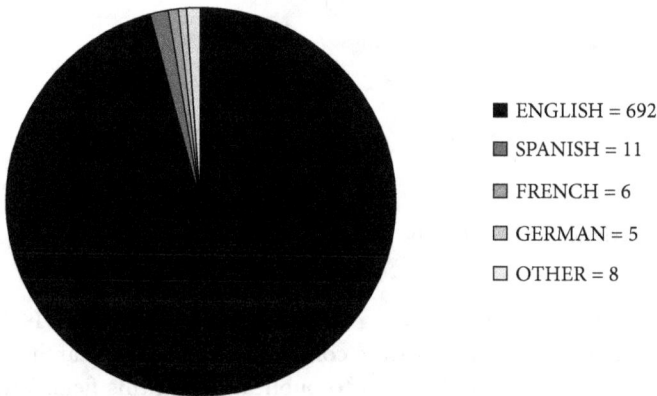

Fig. 3. Distribution of the publications by language

articles (n=306). Other types of publications dealing with the COVID-19 pandemic and human resources in health are letters (n = 176) and editorial material (n = 173). Others are corrections (n=7) and meeting abstracts (n=2).

Fig. 3 shows the distribution of publications by languages. Accordingly, nearly 96 % of the publications are in English. In second and third place, Spanish (n = 11; 1.5 %) and French (n = 6; 0.8 %), respectively. Other languages are Portuguese (n=3), İtalian (n=2), Hungarian (n=1) and Turkish (n=2).

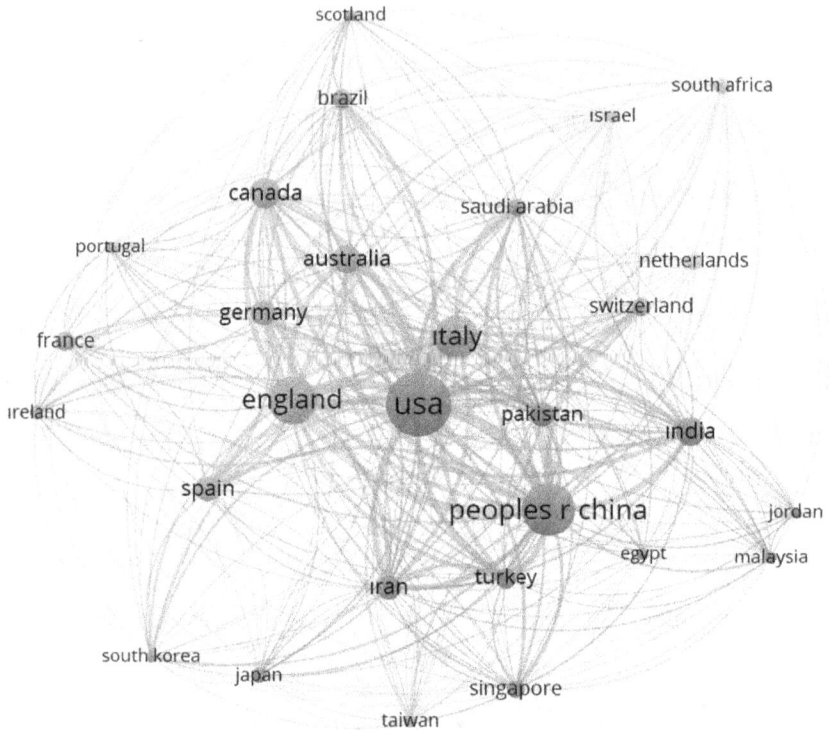

Fig. 4. Countries contributed to the publications

Fig. 4 contains visual information on the countries where COVI9-19 studies on human resources for health were conducted. In total, researchers from 74 different countries have contributed to publications in this field. When these countries are examined in detail, it is seen that studies are rarely conducted in low-income countries and are generally carried out in high and middle-income countries.

Another finding obtained from the study is that the three countries with the most studies are the USA (n=164), People's Republic of China (n=110), and England (n=92). The number of publications is high in Iran and Italy, where diseases and deaths are high. 17 of them originated in Turkey.

Information on the organizations in which the studies on COVID-19 and healthcare professionals were carried out is in Fig. 5. Accordingly, the top three organizations publishing the most publications are Huazhong University

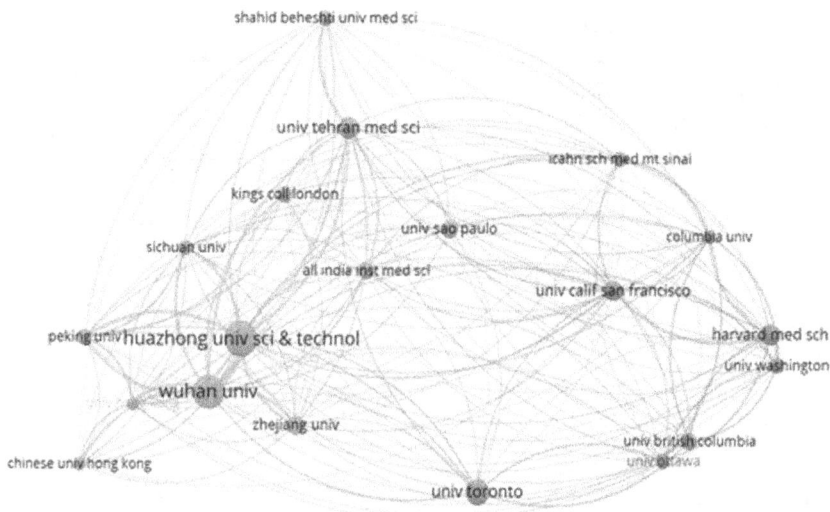

Fig. 5. Distribution of the publications by organizations

Science and Technology (n = 24), Wuhan University and the University of Toronto (n = 15). Huazhong University of Science and Technology (n = 24) and Wuhan University are located in the Wuhan region, where the COVID-19 virus originated in China. The school with the highest number of publications in America is Harvard Medical School with 11 publications in fifth place.

Tab. 1 contains information on the distribution of publications by field of study. According to this, most of the studies are conducted on general internal medicine (n=183; 25.3 %). Public environmental occupational health ranks second. Third place is the studies in the field of nursing. Psychiatry and infectious diseases are two other issues that follow these rankings. When the areas of other studies on COVID and healthcare professionals are examined, it is seen that there are dental, anesthesia and surgeries.

In Fig. 6, there is a visual map of the distribution of the names of the journals in which the studies are published. Accordingly, *BMJ British Medical Journal* (n = 35) is the journal with the most studies on COVID-19 and healthcare personnel. The second and third journals with the highest number of publications are the *International Journal of Environmental Research and Public Health* (n = 21) and *Journal of Hospital Infection* (n = 18), respectively.

Tab. 1. Distribution of publications by study area

Research Area	N	Percent
General Internal Medicine	183	25,3 %
Public Environmental Occupational Health	110	15,2 %
Nursing	65	9,03 %
Psychiatry	62	8,6 %
Infectious Diseases	51	7,1 %
Dentistry Oral Surgery Medicine	45	6,2 %
Health Care Sciences Services	34	4,7 %
Environmental Sciences Ecology	23	3,2 %
Anesthesiology	21	2,9 %
Surgery	21	2,9 %

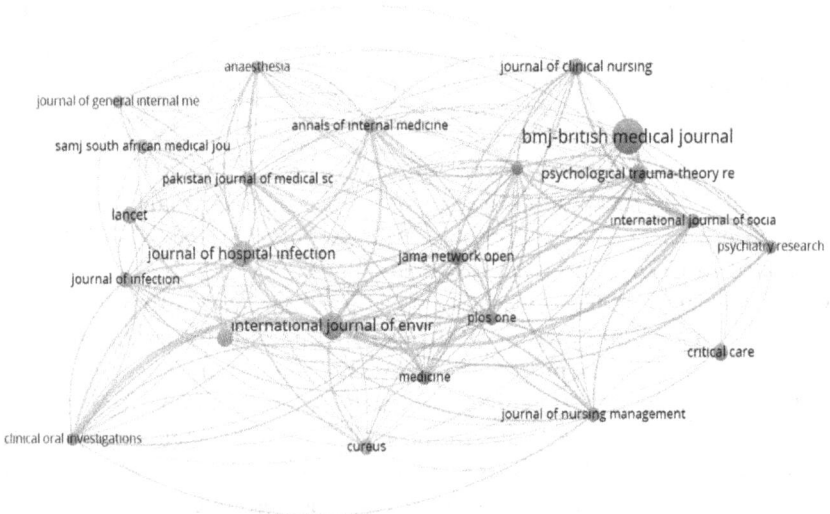

Fig. 6. Distribution of the publications by journals

Tab. 2 contains information on the name, author, journal and number of citations of the first five publications with the most citations. According to the findings obtained from the citation analysis, the most cited publication is the study titled "Factors Associated With Mental Health Outcomes Among Health Care Workers Exposed to Coronavirus Disease 2019" by Lai et al. (2020). This

Tab. 2. Top five publications with the most citations

AUTHOR	TITLE	JOURNAL	CITATION
Lai, Jianbo; Ma, Simeng; Wang, Ying; et al.	Factors Associated With Mental Health Outcomes Among Health Care Workers Exposed to Coronavirus Disease 2019	JAMA NETWORK OPEN	289
Driggin, Elissa; Madhavan, Mahesh V.; Bikdeli, Behnood; et al.	Cardiovascular Considerations for Patients, Health Care Workers, and Health Systems During the COVID-19 Pandemic	JOURNAL OF THE AMERICAN COLLEGE OF CARDIOLOGY	200
Lancet Editor	COVID-19: protecting healthcare workers	LANCET	132
Kang, Lijun; Li, Yi; Hu, Shaohua; et al.	The mental health of medical workers in Wuhan, China dealing with the 2019 novel coronavirus	LANCET PSYCHIATRY	126
Adams, James G.; Walls, Ron M.	Supporting the Health Care Workforce During the COVID-19 Global Epidemic	JAMA-JOURNAL OF THE AMERICAN MEDICAL ASSOCIATION	117

article was published in the Jama Network Open. The number of citations in this article is 289.

Fig. 7 shows the findings regarding the analysis of the keywords in this study. In keyword selection, the condition that the same word should be included in the keywords of at least five different studies was put forward. As a result of the findings obtained, it is seen that the first three most frequently used words in the study are COVID-19 (n = 229), SARS-COV-2 (n = 56) and coronavirus (n = 226), respectively.

When Fig. 7 is examined, it is found that the most frequently used keywords other than COVID and similar words are healthcare workers, personal protective equipment and pandemics. Besides, it is understood from the keywords of the studies that the studies about mental health are more than physical health. Moreover, it is noticed that the studies examining the change in the behavior of healthcare workers towards the organization during the COVID-19 pandemic are very limited, as they are not included in commonly used keywords.

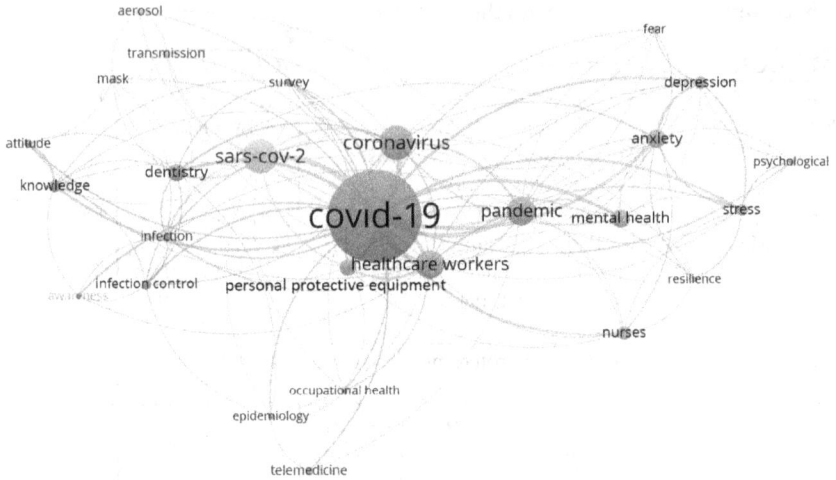

Fig. 7. Co-word analysis results

4. Discussion

COVID-19 has been the world's most critical virus that adversely impacted all facets of life, especially including health and well-being. As governments around the world are making efforts to strengthen health systems to cope with COVID-19, the ongoing epidemic is expected to significantly affect health systems in various dimensions (Etyang, 2020: 9). One of these dimensions, and the most important one, is the healthcare workers fighting on the front lines with the COVID-19 epidemic (Fasogbon et al., 2020: 60). This study aims to provide a general summary of the studies on healthcare workers in the COVID-19 literature with bibliometric analysis.

The first finding obtained from the analysis was that the article was the most preferred study type in this study. 42 % of the studies are articles, and the second most used publication type is letter. In their bibliometric study on COVID, Shamsi et al. (2020) and Dehghanbanadaki et al. (2020) found that articles and letters were the first two most used types of publications. Also, in a bibliometric study conducted by Tsay and Yang (2005), it was found that the most preferred type of document was the article, followed by the letter.

Another finding obtained from the study is that 96 % of the language used in publications is English. This is since English is an official language for many magazines and publishers. As a matter of fact, in a study by Tsay and Yang

(2005), it was determined that 93 % of the publications were in English. Except English, the most used language is Spanish. Ahmi and Mohamad (2019) also stated in their study that Spanish is used as the most second language.

The other finding found in the study is that most of the publications were made in the USA. In a bibliometric study on web access by Ahmi and Mohamad (2019), it was found that most publications were made in America. When examined in terms of countries, it is seen that China is the second most broadcasting country. Similarly, Ellegaard and Wallin (2015) also found that China is the second country that publishes the most. Also, in this study, it was found that there are much fewer studies in developing countries. The results of the bibliometric researches conducted on COVID-19 by Chahrou et al. (2020) and Lou et al. (2020) are consistent with this finding of the study.

When examined in terms of the organization where the research was conducted, it was determined that most of the publications were made in universities in Wuhan. The emergence of the disease in this region is thought to be the reason for the increased intensity of the research. Similary, in the study conducted by Fan et al. (2020) and Hossain (2020), most publications about COVID-19 were made in institutions in China. However, Al-Zaman found that the University of London was the leading institution with the most researches.

In this study, it was determined that the most used keyword was COVID-19. In a bibliometric study conducted by Verma and Gustafsson (2020) in the field of business administration and management, it was found out that the most used co-word was COVID-19 in keyword analysis. Shamsi et al. (2020) also showed that COVID-19 and SARS-COV-2 were the most used two words.

Also, the most researched subject on healthcare professionals is related to mental and psychological problems. Since the fight against COVID-19 began, studies have been found that the prevalence of health problems such as severe anxiety, depression, stress and insomnia among healthcare professionals is relatively high (Itodo et al., 2020: 540; Liu et al., 2020: 790). However, the physical effects of COVID-19 have not been studied much, and it is another phenomenon that affects not only the quality and safety of patient care but also to manage any pandemic (Liu et al., 2020: 790). Therefore, one of the critical priorities for strengthening the readiness of medical personnel to cope with potential emergencies would be to enhance their capacity to deal with physical and mental issues (Fu et al., 2020: 3195).

Another finding found in the keyword analysis in this study is that the behaviors of healthcare workers towards their counsel during their work with COVID-19 have not been adequately investigated. Issues such as job satisfaction, level of commitment, engagement, intention to quit, staff productivity need to be emphasized more than other times in this crisis period. Because all these phenomena can result in staff resignation and leaving the job. Considering the shortage of healthcare personnel around the world, the importance of the issue can be understood much more.

The most vital aspect of this study is that it evaluates past publications with bibliometric analysis. The fact that studies examined by bibliometric methods are not encountered frequently reveals the importance of this study. As a result of this analysis, information is obtained about what kind of studies have been carried out on the subject of interest. Thus, it provides a wide range of current studies and provides more insight into future studies on what kind of gaps still exist.

References

Ahmi, A., & Mohamad, R. (2019). Bibliometric analysis of global scientific literature on Web accessibility. International Journal of Recent Technology and Engineering, 7(6), 250–258.

Al-Zaman. (2020). Bibliometric analysis of COVID-19 literature. Preprints from medRxiv and bioRxiv. doi: https://doi.org/10.1101/2020.07.15.20154989

Bandyopadhyay, S., Baticulon, R. E., Kadhum, M., Alser, M., Ojuka, D. K., Badereddin, Y., ... & Gandino, S. (2020). Infection and mortality of healthcare workers worldwide from COVID-19: A scoping review. MedRxiv, June, 1–37. doi: https://doi.org/10.1101/2020.06.04.20119594

Bartsch, S., Weber, E., Büttgen, M., & Huber, A. (2020). Leadership matters in crisis-induced digital transformation: How to lead service employees effectively during the COVID-19 pandemic. Journal of Service Management. https://doi.org/10.1108/JOSM-05-2020-0160.

Bostan, S., Akbolat, M., Kaya, A., Ozata, M., & Gunes, D. (2020). Assessments of anxiety levels and working conditions of health employees working in COVID-19 pandemic hospitals. Electronic Journal of General Medicine, 17(5), 1–5. https://doi.org/10.29333/ejgm/8228

Buheji, M., da Costa Cunha, K., Beka, G., Mavric, B., de Souza, Y. L., da Costa Silva, S. S., ... & Yein, T. C. (2020). The extent of covid-19 pandemic socio-economic impact on global poverty. A global integrative multidisciplinary review. American Journal of Economics, 10(4), 213–224. doi: 10.5923/j.economics.20201004.02

Burton, J. (2010). WHO healthy workplace framework and model: Background document and supporting literature and practices. Publication of World Health Organization.

Chahrour, M., Assi, S., Bejjani, M., Nasrallah, A. A., Salhab, H., Fares, M., & Khachfe, H. H. (2020). A bibliometric analysis of Covid-19 research activity: A call for increased output. Cureus, 12(3), e7357, 1–8. https://doi.org/10.7759/cureus.7357.

Dehghanbanadaki, H., Seif, F., Vahidi, Y., Razi, F., Hashemi, E., Khoshmirsafa, M., & Aazami, H. (2020). Bibliometric analysis of global scientific research on coronavirus (COVID-19). Medical Journal of The Islamic Republic of Iran (MJIRI), 34(1), 354–362.

Demir, H., & Erigüç, G. (2018). Bibliyometrik bir analiz ile yönetim düşünce sisteminin incelenmesi. İş ve İnsan Dergisi, 5(2), 91–114.

Ellegaard, O., & Wallin, J. A. (2015). The bibliometric analysis of scholarly production: How great is the impact?. Scientometrics, 105(3), 1809–1831.

Etyang, O. (2020). COVID-19 pandemic and its potential impact on the health sector in the COMESA region. Special Report by Common Market for Eastern and Southern Africa.

Fan, J., Gao, Y., Zhao, N., Dai, R., Zhang, H., Feng, X., ... & Bao, S. (2020). Bibliometric analysis on COVID-19: A comparison of research between English and Chinese studies. Frontiers in Public Health, 8, 477.

Fasogbon, S. A., Nnorom, S. C., Fasogbon, L. O., Adebayo, A. O., Omisakin, I. A., Ogunjimi, T. S., ... & Anya, K. K. (2020). COVID-19: The role of welfare and safety of health workers in combating the outbreak. African Journal of Biology and Medical Research, 3(2), 60–65.

Fu, X. W., Wu, L. N., & Shan, L. (2020). Review of possible psychological impacts of COVID-19 on frontline medical staff and reduction strategies. World Journal of Clinical Cases, 8(15), 3188–3196.

Hoffmann, R. L., Battaglia, A., Perpetua, Z., Wojtaszek, K., & Campbell, G. (2020). The clinical nurse leader and COVID-19: Leadership and quality at the point of care. Journal of Professional Nursing, 36(4), 178–180. https://doi.org/10.1016/j.profnurs.2020.06.008

Hossain, M. M. (2020). Current status of global research on novel coronavirus disease (Covid-19): A bibliometric analysis and knowledge mapping. Hossain MM. Current status of global research on novel coronavirus disease (COVID-19): A bibliometric analysis and knowledge mapping. F1000Research 2020, 9:374 https://doi.org/10.12688/f1000research.23690.1

International Labour Organisation (ILO). (2020a). COVID-19 and the health sector. ILO Sectoral Brief.

International Labour Organisation (ILO). (2020b). Managing work-related psychosocial risks during the COVID-19 pandemic. ILO Publications.

Itodo, G. E., Enitan, S. S., Oyekale, A. O., Agunsoye, C. J., Asukwo, U. F., & Enitan, C. B. (2020). COVID-19 among healthcare workers: Risk of exposure, impacts and biosafety measures–A review. International Journal of Health, Safety and Environment, 6(4), 534–548.

Kang, L., Li, Y., Hu, S., Chen, M., Yang, C., Yang, B. X., ... & Chen, J. (2020). The mental health of medical workers in Wuhan, China dealing with the 2019 novel coronavirus. The Lancet Psychiatry, 7(3), 14. https://doi.org/10.1016/S2215-0366(20)30047-X

Kniffin, K. M., Narayanan, J., Anseel, F., Antonakis, J., Ashford, S. J., Bakker, A. B., ... & Creary, S. J. (2020). COVID-19 and the workplace: Implications, issues, and insights for future research and action. Working Paper 20-127, Publication of Harvard Business School. Doi: 10.31234/osf.io/gkwme

Labrague, L. J., & De los Santos, J. A. A. (2020). COVID-19 anxiety among frontline nurses: Predictive role of organisational support, personal resilience and social support. Journal of nursing management, June, 1–9. DOI: 10.1111/jonm.13121

Lai, J., Ma, S., Wang, Y., Cai, Z., Hu, J., Wei, N., ... & Tan, H. (2020). Factors associated with mental health outcomes among health care workers exposed to coronavirus disease 2019. JAMA Network open, 3(3), e203976–e203976.

Lou, J., Tian, S. J., Niu, S. M., Kang, X. Q., Lian, H. X., Zhang, L. X., & Zhang, J. J. (2020). Coronavirus disease 2019: A bibliometric analysis and review. European Review for Medical and Pharmacological Sciences, 24(6), 3411–3421.

Liu, Q., Luo, D., Haase, J. E., Guo, Q., Wang, X. Q., Liu, S., ... & Yang, B. X. (2020). The experiences of healthcare providers during the COVID-19 crisis in China: A qualitative study. The Lancet Global Health, 8, 790–798.

Nemli S., & Demirdal, T. (2016). Ortadoğu solunum yetmezliği sendromu koronavirüsü. Kocatepe Tıp Dergisi, 17(2), 77–83.

Okubo, Y. (1997). Bibliometric indicators and analysis of research systems: Methods and examples. OECD Science, Technology and Industry Working Papers.

Pappa, S., Ntella, V., Giannakas, T., Giannakoulis, V. G., Papoutsi, E., & Katsaounou, P. (2020). Prevalence of depression, anxiety, and insomnia among healthcare workers during the COVID-19 pandemic: A systematic review and meta-analysis. Brain, Behavior, and Immunity, 88, 901–907. https://doi.org/10.1016/j.bbi.2020.05.026

Park, M., Thwaites, R. S., & Openshaw, P. J. (2020). COVID-19: Lessons from SARS and MERS. European Journal of Immunology, 50(3), 308–311.

Peeri, N. C., Shrestha, N., Rahman, M. S., Zaki, R., Tan, Z., Bibi, S., ... & Haque, U. (2020). The SARS, MERS and novel coronavirus (COVID-19) epidemics, the newest and biggest global health threats: what lessons have we learned?. International Journal of Epidemiology, 49(3), 1–10. doi: 10.1093/ije/dyaa033

Petrosillo, N., Viceconte, G., Ergonul, O., Ippolito, G., & Petersen, E. (2020). COVID-19, SARS and MERS: Are they closely related?. Clinical Microbiology and Infection: The official publication of the European Society of Clinical Microbiology and Infectious Diseases, 26(6), 729–734. https://doi.org/10.1016/j.cmi.2020.03.026

Polizzi, C., Lynn, S. J., & Perry, A. (2020). Stress and Coping in the Time of Covid-19: Pathways to Resilience and Recovery. Clinical Neuropsychiatry, 17(2), 59–62. https://doi.org/10.36131/ CN20200204

Rajkumar, R. P. (2020). COVID-19 and mental health: A review of the existing literature. Asian Journal of Psychiatry, 52, 1–6. https://doi.org/10.1016/j.ajp.2020.102066

Shamsi, A., Mansourzadeh, M. J., Ghazbani, A., Khalagi, K., Fahimfar, N., & Ostovar, A. (2020). Contribution of Iran in COVID-19 studies: A bibliometrics analysis. Journal of Diabetes & Metabolic Disorders, 1–10. https://doi.org/10.1007/s40200-020-00606-0

Singhal, T. (2020). A review of coronavirus disease-2019 (COVID-19). The Indian Journal of Pediatrics, 87, 281–286.

Spoorthy, M. S., Pratapa, S. K., & Mahant, S. (2020). Mental health problems faced by healthcare workers due to the COVID-19 pandemic–A review. Asian Journal of Psychiatry, 51, 102119. https://doi.org/10.1016/j.ajp.2020.102119

Sweileh, W. M. (2020). Bibliometric analysis of peer-reviewed literature on climate change and human health with an emphasis on infectious diseases. Globalization and Health, 16, 1–17.

Tsay, M. Y., & Yang, Y. H. (2005). Bibliometric analysis of the literature of randomized controlled trials. Journal of the Medical Library Association, 93(4), 450.

Tuncay, F. E., Koyuncu, E., & Özel, Ş. (2020). Pandemilerde sağlık çalışanlarının psikosoyal sağlığını etkileyen koruyucu ve risk faktörlerine ilişkin bir derleme. Ankara Medical Journal, 2, 488–501. Doi:10.5505/amj.2020.02418

Wang, J., Zhou, M., & Liu, F. (2020). Reasons for healthcare workers becoming infected with novel coronavirus disease 2019 (COVID-19) in China. Journal of Hospital Infection, 1051, 1–2. https://doi.org/10.1016/j.jhin.2020.03.002 0195-6701

Wei, G. (2019). A bibliometric analysis of the top five economics journals during 2012–2016. Journal of Economic Surveys, 33(1), 25–59.

Verma, S., & Gustafsson, A. (2020). Investigating the emerging COVID-19 research trends in the field of business and management: A bibliometric analysis approach. Journal of Business Research, 118, 253–261. https://doi.org/10.1016/j.jbusres.2020.06.057

World Health Organization. (2020a). Coronavirus disease 2019 (COVID-19): Situation report, 208. Publication of World Health Organization.

World Health Organization. (2020b). Protocol for assessment of potential risk factors for coronavirus disease 2019 (COVID-19) among health workers in a health care setting. Publication of World Health Organization.

World Trade Organization. (2020). Trade in services in the context of COVID-19. Publication of World Trade Organization.

Wu, Y., Wang, J., Luo, C., Hu, S., Lin, X., Anderson, A. E., ... & Qian, Y. (2020). A comparison of burn-out frequency among oncology physicians and nurses working on the front lines and usual wards during the COVID-19 epidemic in Wuhan, China. Journal of Pain and Symptom Management, 60(1), e60–e65. https://doi.org/10.1016/j.jpainsymman.2020.04.008

Zaki, N., Alashwal, H., & Ibrahim, S. (2020). Association of hypertension, diabetes, stroke, cancer, kidney disease, and high-cholesterol with COVID-19 disease severity and fatality: A systematic review. Diabetes & Metabolic Syndrome, 14(5), 1133–1142. Advance online publication. https://doi.org/10.1016/j.dsx.2020.07.005

Zhou, M., Yuan, F., Zhao, X., Xi, F., Wen, X., Zeng, L., ... & Zhao, Z. (2020). Research on the individualized short-term training model of nurses in emergency isolation wards during the outbreak of COVID-19. Nursing Open, 1–7. DOI: 10.1002/nop2.580

Zupic, I., & Čater, T. (2015). Bibliometric methods in management and organization. Organizational Research Methods, 18(3), 429–472.

www.ingramcontent.com/pod-product-compliance
Lightning Source LLC
Chambersburg PA
CBHW050655280326
41932CB00015B/2923